DIETS AND OTHER UNNATURAL ACTS

Stewart B Segal, M.D. &
Barbara M. Phillips, Ph.D.

9/17/2011

Copyright © 2011 Stewart Barry Segal M.D. & Barbara M Phillips Ph.D.
All rights reserved.

ISBN: 061553807X
ISBN-13: 9780615538075
Library of Congress Control Number: 2011938757
CreateSpace, North Charleston, SC

TABLE OF CONTENTS

Dr Segal's Dedication

To the tens of thousands of patients, families, and generations of families who have walked through the doors of Lake Zurich Family Treatment Center and to those who will walk through our doors in the years to come

And

To my children, Lisa, Jeremy, Erin, Tim, and Allyson who heard about this book for years and always thought it was another one of my pipedreams

Dr Phillips's Dedication

To my sons, Mark and Ray, and my brothers, Webb and Peter, all of whom have contributed to it more than they realize

INTRODUCTION

Make no mistake. **Wellthy** is not a diet book. I hate diets! Instead, what you will find here is a philosophy of life born from thirty years of practicing family medicine. During that time, I've witnessed hundreds of fad diets, exercise routines, and high tech equipment come and go. My patients have lost thousands of pounds, only to gain them back, often gaining more than what they had lost. Not only did this seesaw effect damage their health, every failure made it that much more difficult to succeed. Every failure left them frustrated and depressed. Other people lose weight, so why can't I?

Not only did failures result in an overall weight gain, some diets caused measurable physical harm. Meanwhile, the diet craze continues; treadmills and exercycles gather dust. New diets hit the market almost daily and old diets are reborn. We quickly forget our bad experiences. We are who we are and changing ourselves is difficult. Because most diets demand that we become someone else for a while, we steal from ourselves, we deny and deprive ourselves, and often we lie to ourselves. We tell ourselves we can't eat this or that or the other, and we promise we will never return to our old ways of eating.

We set short-term goals for long-term problems until old habits pull us back. As we falter, we feel hopeless and alone. As our despair increases, we eat. The cycle starts all over again.

As a family physician, one of my most important tools is to communicate with my patients in a manner they can understand and incorporate into their daily lives. Since I started practicing, I have used analogies as a primary method of communicating. Saving for our financial retirement seems a useful analogy for saving our health. Here is where **WELLTHY** comes in.

Wellth is not a misspelled word! It's a new concept that stems from a critical lesson my patients have taught me. I live and practice in an affluent suburb of Chicago where many of my patients are financially wealthy at the expense of their health. No matter how much money you accumulate, if you don't have your health, you don't have anything. Yet millions of people trade their lives for money. They save for tomorrow, for tomorrow they will have it all. Tomorrow they will have the money to retire, buy their dream home, and play golf any time they please. There is a critical fallacy in their reasoning. The problem is that, very often, when they finally retire, either their health or their marriage fails. There are lots of retirees with plenty of money who are neither healthy nor happy. **Wellthy** is about investing in your physical, nutritional, emotional, and spiritual selves. **Wellthy** is about setting long-term goals and plotting a slow, steady course to reaching them.

I believe in promoting health with preventative medicine. Unfortunately, we don't have a health care system in this country; we have a sick care system. Most people come to me looking for a quick fix. Something is broken and they want it repaired. Over the last 30 years, I've done a lot of repairs. I've come to understand that illness is an imbalance in one or in several components of an individual's life. These components are one's physical, nutritional, emotional, financial, and spiritual well-being. We have wellth when we've achieved balance among all these areas of life. Here's where my analogy fits in.

Most of us understand the concept of a financial retirement fund. We either have one or we want one. Retirement funds employ long-term planning to meet long-term goals. They are successful when we make small, regular deposits into them over a long period of time. We don't need to deprive ourselves of anything substantial to build them. Since our goals are long-term, failures are rare. Can you imagine what would happen if your life depended on your depositing $1,000,000.00 in a retirement fund in 3 months? You would have to rob banks! Even if you were able to pull it off, you'd spend the rest of your life paying for it, either in jail time and fines or running and waiting to get caught. Deciding to lose 30 pounds in 90 days is very much like robbing the bank. It's no wonder we gain 45 pounds back. Deciding to run 6 miles today when you have not exercised in 3 years is equally foolhardy. Deciding, instead, that you want to run in a marathon and then spending months training (investing in one's self) to build strength and endurance is much more rational.

One of the greatest privileges of being a family physician is the opportunity to meet such a broad spectrum of individuals. All of them have helped me formulate the idea of wellth. Many have road tested this concept and improved their lots in life. They have joined our 200 Club and established "Life Savings Accounts."

Life Savings Account and the 200 Club

Now that you are becoming familiar with the concept of "Wellth," it's time for you to think about establishing your own "Life Savings Account." What is your Life Savings Account? I want you to think about your physical, emotional, nutritional, and spiritual selves the way you think about your finances, as if you had accounts for each at the local bank. You can make deposits and withdrawals into these additional accounts. Most people are born with their physical and emotional accounts fully vested. Ever see a baby smile, coo, or hear him laugh? His emotional account is full. As we age, we spend those assets. Illness, injury, and neglect subtract physical assets. Life, in general, fills and depletes our emotional accounts. Our nutritional and spiritual accounts are developed by our family, religion, and the society in which we live. **WELLTHY** will help you discover how to make deposits in all of your health accounts.

Read on to learn about the **200 Club.** Membership requires investments in self. Through little investments, 200 calories or 200 seconds, **LIVING WELLTHY** enriches you. To start you on your journey, I want to introduce you to the twins.

Raucous Ralph and his identical twin, So-so Sam, were born 62 years ago. Their mother died at the age of 64 from the effects of diabetes and hypertension. She was pleasingly plump, thriving on meat, potatoes, salt, and chocolate. Their father had his first heart attack at 48, a second at 52, and died from a stroke at 62. He was a big man who ate, drank, and smoked too much.

The boys were raised to eat! They celebrated birthdays with cake, holidays with childhood treats, days ending in "y" with deep fried food orgies. So-so Sam played sports. Ralph partied hearty. I met them later in life. So-so first came to me when he was 48. He was worried because his folks died young and he decided it was time to get his health in order. His brother met me in the Emergency Room 2 years ago. He was having his first heart attack.

When So-so first came to my office, he was working as a stockbroker. He was making a good living and had saved substantial funds. He smoked ¾ of a pack of cigarettes a day, had 10 cocktails a week, and described his life as stressful. He had 4 children and a lovely wife he often argued with. While he tried to exercise, his efforts always failed. He got winded climbing one flight of stairs. The last time he went to church was Christmas Eve, 3 years ago. For fun, he took naps. His life was so-so.

So-so Sam's life savings account looked like:

Financial

- $200,000 in stocks, bonds, etc.
- $600,000 house with $425,000 mortgage
- $10,000 in bank
- Leased cars
- College savings account of $35,000

He had a firm plan to increase his assets and knew exactly what he wanted to have in the bank when he retired at 65 years old. He had this part of his life in order.

Physical

- 5 feet 10 inches and 250 pounds of poorly distributed fat, some muscle
- Blood pressure was 165/96 (elevated)
- Short of breath when playing kickball with his 5 year old son
- Infrequent intimacy with his wife due to shortness of breath and pounding pulse
- Blood sugar borderline, cholesterol elevated
- Smoking ¾ pack a day; he denied coughing; his wife stated he coughs every morning; he countered that morning cough is due to his allergies

He's hypertensive and soon to be diabetic. You could give good odds that his heart attack was imminent. His physical account was bankrupt!

Nutritional

- Sugar in ice cream, sugar cookies, candy, and chocolate, chocolate on ice cream; So-so was not so-so when it came to the consumption of sugar!
- Fried ice cream, fried anything in mass quantity!
- Alcohol in abundance, with country fried steak and greasy French fries; So-so liked everything he shouldn't
- No vegetables, no fiber, an occasional piece of fruit (usually banana in banana split)

Needless to say, So-so Sam's nutritional account was poorly invested in risky junk food markets and on the verge of collapse.

Emotional

- 1 hour commute to 12 hour job to 1 hour commute back home left no time for fun
- Weekend life revolved around moving kids from here to there to everywhere
- Strained relationship with wife who wants a little attention from her husband
- Kids have "I-want-it" dis-ease
- Performance at work suffering and prospect for promotion is so-so

Emotional account is OK because Sam is too busy and too tired to notice that he is unhappy, stressed, and on his way to depression.

Spiritual

- No time for church
- Goes to kids' religious events
- Sleeps late Sundays

So-so Sam awoke on his 48th birthday with a pang of fear. He had gotten old and he didn't like what he saw in the mirror. His wife made an appointment for a full physical exam and Sam started his journey. When I reviewed his asset list, I thought he was going to keel over. Instead, he took the first step by asking, "What can I do? Is it too late?" That began the process. I introduced Sam to the Wellthy concept as follows:

1. Define the problems
2. Set new goals
3. Refine, polish, and improve yourself.

Financial

Sam worried about the future of his job and started looking at other options. He wanted a "Timewrap" (see Appendix A) that would give him financial security while cutting his commute and work hours.

Physical

Sam was tired of being overweight and out of shape. He wanted to lose weight, increase stamina and strength, and learn to breathe again. He wanted to make love to his wife without having a heart attack. He wanted to get off the cigarettes but was sure he couldn't because he'd tried before and failed.

Nutritional

While Sam knew change was essential to his well-being, he did not want to change. Food was his love, his solace, and his only real happiness. We negotiated and, after a while, came up with the following goals: fresh, nutritionally-laden food balancing low fat and reduced sugar options. He agreed to consume less alcohol and add more veggies. Once Sam understood the concept of "chicken steps," he became more comfortable with the goals he set.

(One of the first jokes I learned was, "How did the chicken get to the other side of the road?" The answer was

"Chicken-steps," one tiny step at a time. By taking small steps, one after another, toward his goals, he, or you or anyone, can attain wellth.)

Emotional

This was the easiest to work on. Sam wanted to re-discover his wife. He missed her. His first goal was to send the kids to his brother's and run away with his wife. He decided that 14-hour days were killing him and paralyzing his relationships. He also really liked the concept of "self" time.

Spiritual

Sam placed this item on the back burner. By recognizing how far he had strayed from his beliefs, he had at least defined where he currently was and, in time, would start the refining process.

Chicken steps have carried Sam to where he is today. Physically, he is much improved. He began exercising 10 minutes a day, which became 15, then 20, and now 60. He walks, uses an elliptical machine, and lifts weights. He is still overweight but now weighs in at 225 and has improved his body fat ratio by 8%. He can play kickball with his children and grandchildren without being winded. His wife no longer worries that he'll die making love, to her that is. It took Sam 6 years of hard work to stop smoking and his work has paid off. His "normal" morning cough is now a thing of the past.

Sam works as a consultant now. He recreated his career shortly after his 49th birthday. He spends lots of time at home, traveling only 2 days a week. His finances are good and he's happy with his work and soon to retire.

Eating is still his nemesis. He still loves food but food is no longer his only joy and solace. His chicken steps were really tiny and he is still on his journey. From ½ quart of Ben and Jerry's Phish to a 3-ounce scoop was a journey that took years. How long it took to get there was not as important as the fact that he finally arrived. His French fry technique is worth reporting. On the way to the table, Sam would throw 5 fries out, and then devour his "Biggie" fry. Once he realized that he did not need those 5 fries, he started chucking 10, then 15. Now, Sam occasionally buys a regular size bag of fries and throws out 10. He's delighted with the remainder.

Sam's spiritual account was jerked to the front with the death of a dear cousin. If you were to ask him what he would do differently knowing what he knows now, Sam would say that he would have respected his life sooner.

When I first saw him in the emergency room, Sam's brother, Raucous Ralph, looked bad. He had totally abused his body. A big man, weighing in at more than 300 pounds, he was pale and sweaty. His pain was decreasing but he had a headache from the nitroglycerin drip and was throwing up from the morphine. At 62, his life savings account was on empty.

Despite the pain and drugs, Ralph was still a stitch. His keen sense of humor was his strongest asset. He often boasted that he was a skinny person trapped in a fat body. He claimed to have lost 300 pounds in his lifetime. Raucous Ralph did everything big. He went on every popular diet, becoming the poster child for healthy eating, but only for a while. Trouble is, he always reverted to the real Ralph, and Ralph ate just like his brother used to. Ralph would never chicken step. Ironically, he was always trying to get his brother to go on this fad diet, that fad diet, or the other fad diet. He didn't chicken step to finance either. Ralph boasted that he's been a millionaire 6 times over. Unfortunately, he's lost it all 7 times. Ralph's rushing to success has always prevented his success.

Ralph always buys the latest exercise equipment. He sprained his ankle on the treadmill, his back on the weight bench, and injured his groin on the bike. He doesn't work-out consistently because he feels that he's "accident-prone." If only he had eased into a routine.

Ralph felt very alone in the E.R. His second divorce ended badly and the kids are estranged. He felt that he's been unlucky in love. Ralph never invested in himself or others and the cost to his body and self has been tremendous.

Following Ralph's discharge from the hospital, he promised to work on his Life Savings Account. His brother is trying to teach him the chicken step concept. Ralph grasps concepts slowly, but there is hope.

Your life is a precious gift. It's time to get to work building your accounts. It's easy. Define where you are today. Dare to dream where you would like to be 1, 5, 10, 20 years from now. Establish your Life Savings Accounts and start making any deposits you can. See your financial advisor to answer your money questions. See your doctor to evaluate your other assets. Study your family history as it will help show you the future. You can change the future if you are willing to put in the time to do so. It takes a little work and a lot of **chicken steps**.

In the Beginning

It's the New Year. You resolve to diet tomorrow. For sure! Tomorrow you will feast on tofu lumps and carrot chunks and swear off nachos for the entire millennium. Never again will a chocolate éclair or an ice-cold beer greet your lips. At dinner, you will munch on fricassee of algae while dishing up crispy fried chicken for the family. When you go out to eat, you'll graze on cauliflower and kale stalks, oblivious to the ambient aroma of sizzling sirloin and the mouthwatering sight of the chocolate truffles at the next table. In the evening, you'll sip your second gallon of water for the day while you catch the news, the weather report, and the commercials for juicy burgers with cheese fries. You'll quit smoking, give up the booze, and never cuss again.

As for exercise, you'll sign up for triathlons and join the local boxing gym. No more driving to work. You'll park the car 5 miles away so that you can sprint through the crowds, perfecting your jumping jacks as you go. You'll leap up the stairs, 2 at a time, to your 10th floor office, skip down the hall to the water cooler, and practice squats at your desk. After work, it's off to aerobics class before you race home to pedal to Peoria on your exercise bike. Tomorrow! Absolutely! Positively! You are looking forward to it as much as having a root canal except root canals are quicker.

You'll run away with your wife, go to Paris, even make love from dusk to dawn. When you get back, you'll take the kids to Disney. Since you are going to be fit, you'll climb Mount Everest. You'll do everything you've ever dreamed of, tomorrow! Today, you'll work to pay for it.

Today is the day you make a killing in the market! You'll quit your job, buy expensive cars and houses. You'll spend a few hours a day managing your funds. Today is the day! You would pray on it if you had not forgotten how.

This book isn't about dieting because diets are cruel and unusual punishment and we don't like them either. Nor must you press hundreds of pounds or climb to Mars on your Stairmaster. **WELLTHY** is about investing in your health the same way you save money so that you can retire in comfort and indulge in activities you've waited all your life to do. It applies the principles of successful investing to help you balance your body like you balance your checkbook. In fact, using a check register from the bank is one of the best ways to track your debits and credits as you earn and lose your bucks (points). These principles work just as well for your body as they do for your money and you are probably already acquainted, if not downright friendly, with them. **WELLTHY** will teach you to **define** goals, and then **refine** your habits and "self" in order to reach those goals. We will teach you to **chicken step** your way to **wellth**, one tiny step at a time. We will show you how to join the **200 Club** and save for your future wellth much as you have saved for years in your Christmas account.

Diets and Other Unnatural Acts hasn't a single recipe for bean sprout barbecue, seaweed taffy, or anything else that makes you gag. We want you to enjoy your meals because, sooner or later, everyone eats what s/he likes; and we have no intention of making you a guilt-ridden wreck, gobbling cookies in the dark. Nor will we attempt to force you to abandon foods that bring you more pleasure than winning the lottery. We will encourage you to improve your wellness skills doing activities you like and to practice them when and where you prefer. Notice that we said activity, not exercise. The word "exercise" leaves a bad taste in the mouths of many of us who can't get excited about weightlifting and wall climbing, pastimes that are obviously designed to kill us. We will encourage you to spend more "**self**" time, as well as quality time, with those you love. Establishing an emotional account and making regular investments will be critical to your success.

Ease is an essential concept we want you to get comfortable with. The dictionary defines ease as "Freedom from difficulty, hardship, or effort." What a marvelous concept it is! With "ease," there is much you can accomplish. We will teach you about Financ-ease, Food-ease, Fit-ease, Self-ease, and Dis-ease, concepts created so that you can be eased into health and wellth. Remember, Chicken steps are easy, small steps.

By following a few simple investment principles, you'll grow both financially wealthy and rich in mind, body, and spirit. All you need do is invest systematically in small amounts, for as long as it takes to reach the goals you've set for yourself. Doing so earns dividends that compound over time, paying you greater and greater returns the longer you keep at it. You are free to choose investments that fit your style and to refine and diversify them to balance your wellthy portfolio. Your unique self-ness, soul, spirit, or whatever you want to call it, is the core of wellth. It, too, deserves your attention because it pays handsome returns on your efforts. Please turn the page to start becoming a real-life millionaire with true wellth.

CHAPTER 1.
FINANCE-EASE

Let's begin!

I want to be a millionaire. YES____ NO____ (If you say no, quit reading.)

I will spend my first million doing these things:

1. ____

2. ____

3. ____

(You can write in this book and won't be sent to the principal's office.)

Think big. I'll cruise the Caribbean, build a cabin in Colorado, or buy a condo in Maui. At the very least, I'll have the million in personal investments that many financial planners predict I'll need to live comfortably in 2020.

When Frugal Frank and Patient Patty were 21, they began stashing $4.00 a day ($2.00 each) in their respective 401k plans at work. Over the years, their tax-deferred investments paid 6 to 10 %, on the $120.00 per month ($60.00 apiece) their employers deducted from their paychecks. At age 65, they are millionaires enjoying the good life hiking in the Swiss Alps and skiing at Aspen, with a paid-up mortgage and no debts. For the price of a cup of coffee and a donut every day, they guaranteed their prosperity for life. It doesn't take an MBA to figure out that, when you save day after day, year after year, you positively will get rich.

It is fun to illustrate your dream list with pictures cut from magazines or newspapers. (Be a diplomat and include your partner's dreams, too, unless he/she wants to retire to a cave in Greenland.) If you lust after a certain Cessna or Corvette, find photos of them. Look in the real estate sections of Sunday newspapers for images of glamorous homes and in the travel sections for idyllic beach scenes. Golf nuts should search for photos of their favorite courses; bass fishing devotees can hunt for pictures of the perfect lake. If you prefer trekking the Andes or white water rafting, snip images of glorious mountain peaks or sparkling West Virginia river rapids. Your pictorial dream list is a variation on the "What will I do when I win the lottery" game most people play without specifying what they would do because they don't expect to win.

To jump-start your new million, even if you have other investments, stash 200 cents in a jar today and every day, every week and month for 365 days. Well, almost every day. Skipping a day is OK as long as you make up for it the next. Encourage the kids to put their 200 cents worth in their own jars by threatening to cut off their entire allowance until they comply. Label the jars, "Do not disturb, Millions at work," and try not to rob them or fondle their contents too much.

In a couple of weeks, you'll have $28.00; in a month, $60.00 (unless it's February). Your goal is to hoard 72,000 cents ($720.00) a year, plus interest. Once a month, transfer your stashes to an IRA or other instrument that accepts contributions of this size and wait for your money to bloom.

You may protest, "But I can't afford to save $2.00 a day. I need my money now to pay my mortgage, my property taxes, my car payments." Pull two dollar bills out of your wallet and ask yourself, "Must I spend this today? Can I keep it by bringing my coffee, tea, or soda from home instead of buying it at work? Could I whip up dinner from scratch tonight instead of paying for carryout? Should I check out that hot CD or DVD from the library rather than buying it?" These are the small changes that can make you rich.

"How?," Dr. P once asked her secretary, an astute Indiana native, "am I going to get all my work done?"

"In CHICKEN STEPS," said Lucy. Tiny steps, trivial steps that mean nothing in themselves, yet many strung together lead to success.

To take your first chicken step on the million-dollar highway, grab a pencil and calculate your present investments.

My Money Investments Now

Name of Plan $ Amount currently invested

401k/403b ______________________________

Pension ______________________________

IRA ________________________________

Keogh/SEP ________________________________

403s/Simple ________________________________

Other: CDs, T-bill, and etc. ________________

Value of my home/s less mortgage/s ____________

Total investments ________________________

The first 3 apply to people working for someone else, the next 2 to self-employed persons. If you aren't taking advantage of your employer's 401k plan (403b if your employer is a not-for-profit organization such as a school), run, don't walk, to sign up. Most 401ks are the investment choice of the 21st century because they allow you to invest in small, but frequent, tax-deferred increments.

Next, calculate your earnings from each of your investments. Your plan administrator at work can tell you what your 401k is earning, as can her counterparts for your IRAs and other instruments. Let's say you invested in 3 of the mutual funds offered by your plan. These funds are currently returning an average of 8%. At this rate, if you are 30 years old, you will need to invest $300.00 every month to grow a million at age 67.

Whoa! That's a bunch of dough! It's $10.00 a day to be exact. To improve your returns, you can switch to funds paying 12%, funds that might be riskier but they will cost less per month. The quickest route to riches is to start early as Frank and Patty did because the younger you are when you begin, the faster your investments will grow. At age 45, you need $760.00 a month at earnings of 15% a year to garner a million in 20 years.

That's fine for you, you may be thinking; but I don't know anything about the stock market. Besides, playing the lottery is more fun. Join the crowd. Most of us don't understand stocks, bonds, REITs, or various other financial instruments. We need an advisor to help us choose investments appropriate to our goals. The managers of our 401k plans, bank personnel, and personal financial planners can give us a hand. The funds they represent usually are far safer than sinking your money in the lottery where you have about as much chance of winning big as you have of being attacked by a band of crazed armadillos.

True horror stories abound about people losing their shirts investing in oil futures, pork bellies, and Death Valley real estate. All investments carry risks, from extremely high risks, such as acreage on Saturn, to extremely low-risk instruments, such as bank CDs or T-bills. The trade-off is that high-risk products may pay handsome returns, while low-risk ones pay peanuts. What to do? Ask yourself, am I a high-risk, "all-or-none" gambler or a cautious, "don't waste a dime" miser? Choose investments that don't give you nightmares, but remember that none is 100% guaranteed to make money. If you never leave your home, you won't be killed in an automobile accident, though you may slip while feeding your pet alligator and become his next meal. Unless the US government collapses, you won't lose sleep or money by stashing your bucks in savings bonds and treasury bills. You won't get rich either because your earnings will barely keep pace with inflation. The kinds of instruments in which you invest illustrate your style, meaning your attitudes toward spending. One person's style may be to day trade on the Internet, while someone else may prefer mutual funds. Regardless of your style, it's smart to spread your money among different kinds of products, for example, bonds, mutual funds, stocks, certificates of deposit, and real estate. When you DIVERSIFY your investments this way, you maximize your possibilities for gain and minimize your potential for losses. This extremely important strategy, called BALANCING your portfolio, is what most investors in their right minds do.

Confident Connie, age 35, has her employer withhold 5% of her annual salary of $40,000 for her 401k plan. Her employer then matches 4%, or $1600.00 of her salary for a total investment of $3600.00 per year. She invests 70% in stocks and 30% in bonds paying an average of 10% in dividends and interest, all of which she reinvests. With each raise, she saves more money without having to up the percentage she invests. Connie knows for sure that she will be worth a million at age 65. What makes her so cocky? She remembers what Albert Einstein said: "COMPOUNDING is the 8th wonder of the world." Like rabbits, your investments beget more money each year in interest and/or dividends -begetting which never ends so long as you reinvest your earnings. If you invest $1000.00 a year in an instrument earning 10%, obviously, you will have $1100.00 at the end of the first year. Keep it up for 7 years and your annual earnings will exceed your annual deposit of $1000.00. In a few more years, your investment earnings will be double the amount of your yearly contribution. A few years later, your earnings will triple your annual contribution. This is the ultimate payoff for your sacrifices because it's "free" money, money that multiplies without you raising a finger to earn it. Compounding is the dividend you pocket for chicken-stepping your way to wealth. If the idea means nothing to you because you spend all your money before it hits your wallet, check your:

Spending Habits

Yes

No

1. I was born to shop.

___

___

2. Money burns holes in my pocket.

___

___

3. When I see something I like, I want it Now.

___

___

4. I can't get out of a store for less than $200.00.

___

___

5. There's no money left after I pay the bills.

___

___

6. I like to buy nice things for my family & friends, not for me.

___

___

7. I'll save money later.

___

___

8. I try to save but there is always something I need.

___

___

9. I'm too busy to think about investments.

___

___

10. Other____

___

___

The way you spend mirrors your feelings about finances, feelings that, in turn, reflect the attitudes of your parents, spouse, friends, and business associates. Maybe money was the bone your parents constantly fought over; or, perhaps as a child, you learned that, when you wheedled, begged and told a few lies, you could get daddy to buy you whatever you wanted. Most partners include a Rockefeller who isn't troubled by unpaid bills and hefty interest charges on credit cards and a Scrooge who counts every nickel twice and spends weeks ferreting out the cheapest toilet paper. This mismatch between partners accounts for more discord than having sex or any other topic, for the simple reason that the participants have completely different financial styles. Make your motto "DEFINE and REFINE" and think about the spending goals you listed on the first page. "Defining" is what you did when you listed your current assets. "Refining" is making the small changes in your spending that will allow you to realize your dreams. You can define and refine any lifestyle and maybe even compromise with a partner whose spending habits drive you crazy.

For instance, High-roller Hiram loved trying to beat the house odds in Vegas. He would rather give up his wife than gambling. She disagreed, loudly and incessantly. To keep the peace, he now makes 2 trips to Vegas a year instead of the 6 he used to take and tosses the moola he used to drop at the casinos into the stock market. Last year, he reaped the dividends of a happier wife and a modest profit by trading shares on the Internet. Hiram knew he couldn't give up gambling, though he wanted to save for retirement and stay married, too. He refined his spending by switching from craps to stocks; since playing the market satisfies his need to bet, he doesn't feel deprived of his favorite pastime.

If you love a bargain, frequent thrift shops and garage sales for the ultimate in cheap recycling, visit the library to test new games, draw terrific graphics for greeting cards, borrow a movie or attend a family storytelling session. (Libraries also lend books.) Another chicken step to investing is to brown bag your work lunches. Packing your lunch will save at least $5.00 a day ($1,000.00 a year) if you normally spend

$7.50 for fast food. Eating carryout pizza or Chinese once instead of twice a week saves another $500.00 or more. Instead of swearing off surf and turf forever, prepare a vegetarian meal from scratch once a week. Invite the family to cook vegetable lasagna or pizza or tacos and pocket your meatless savings. Think generics, store brands, and sale items at the supermarket. Sip lemonade, not soda, and microwave your own popcorn and potato chips in place of expensive store-bought brands.

Camping in the backyard for a week of your vacation saves another grand. Buying special occasion clothes at designer discount stores and discovering quality furniture at resale shops or on-line auctions contributes a bit more. Serious savers can try swap and barter. When you travel, swap your house for someone else's on the coast of Spain or host travelers in your home who will then host you in theirs. An interior decorator we know barters her services for baby-sitting, massages, dentistry, and computer programming while she increases her business exposure. Combining a few of these money saving ideas gets you an almost-free IRA that generates even more savings. Discovering these chicken steps to investments is as much fun as stumbling upon bargains at a flea market. An occasional frivolous buy is a fine reward for being a loyal 200 Club member. Besides, it feels good.

To ease the pain of saving money, avoid your triggers to unproductive spending. Jot down a list of essentials before you hit the mall or the Internet. Milk for the kids is essential; a rhinestone collar for the iguana is not. Carry limited cash (no credit cards) in your pockets to shop for things you need, not the ones you buy to feel better. Before you shell out your money, ask yourself, "Do I crave this cashmere coat or power drill or box of Godiva because I'm bored? Stressed? Buying makes me feel powerful?" If so, hide your credit cards before you hit the mall or surf the Internet. When you spot an incredible bargain, take a deep breath and a brisk walk until the feeling passes–unless it's a once-in-a-lifetime, not-to-be believed steal at any price. If it is, jump on it.

Financ-ease is taking charge of your income in the style you choose. It is knowing you deserve the time and attention you spend researching your investments and maybe gloating a bit that you are such a financial genius. Decide how much you must stash to accrue a million in 20 or 30 years, or whenever you plan to take up permanent residence on Samoa. Then, arrange to have this amount deducted from your paycheck or checking account every month because money you never see is infinitely easier to save than cash in the hand. A fun exercise is to calculate the tax savings on your investments. For instance, if you move $2000.00 a year to a tax-deferred IRA and your federal taxes are 20%, you save $400.00 a year. That's $1.10 a day to feed to your 200 Club.

Let's recap the chicken steps to financ-ease:

1. Choose to be rich and stick to your decision.
2. **DEFINE** your financial goals.
3. Assess your present financial condition.
4. Join Club 200.
5. **REFINE** your spending to meet your goals.
6. Seek guidance from an advisor.
7. Choose investments that suit your style.

8. **DIVERSIFY** your investments for maximum returns.
9. **BALANCE** your portfolio.
10. Assess your portfolio regularly and revise it as your needs change.

Get ready to discover how these steps work every bit as well for investing in your health as they do for your savings accounts. Maybe better.

CHAPTER 2. WHAT IS WELLTH?

Workaholic Willy was a successful trade magazine publisher with a net worth of $5 million, give or take a couple hundred thousand. His business was his life, whether conducted at his city office, his penthouse overlooking Lake Michigan, or his beachfront home north of Malibu. He paid no attention to his weakening body, his 4 martini lunches with colleagues, or his 2-pack a day smoking habit. Telling people they were vitamins, he gulped tranquilizers by the fistful and washed them down with a nip from the bottle in his bottom drawer. When he sold his business at a huge profit, he was so sick he spent most of his time in doctor's offices and hospitals. He figured he could buy his way out of clogged arteries, kidney malfunction, and liver failure, just as he had always bought his way out of business problems. He couldn't. He died at the age of 67, leaving his estate to his wife and kids. They didn't want his money. They wanted Willy.

Willy isn't an extreme case. Like many of us, he measured success solely with a financial yardstick, completely disregarding any balance between earning a living and living. It's easy to believe that financial wealth is a bubbling hot tub of happiness that will soak us in happiness because money is real. We see it, smell it, and fondle it. We can buy a Jaguar with it. Our problems would vanish if we had a little more of it. The authors suggest that a fit and healthy body, rich in panache and passion, rather than financial wealth, defines success. It isn't healthy to hurtle down the expressway cutting off every car you can and cursing and tailgating the others. Driving with a cell phone in one hand, while taking notes with the other, is not good exercise. Your life isn't balanced when all you do is work and chauffeur the kids or when your conversations with your spouse consist of "Pass the salt, please," and "Did you pay the gas bill?" At the very least, good health is essential to enjoying your financial investments. Are you going to get your money's worth?

Larcenous Larry decided he just had to invest a hundred thou in some "can't lose" futures. Since he could not possibly earn that much money in a hurry, he embezzled it from his employer. He got caught. After paying his lawyers and fines forced him into bankruptcy, he had plenty of free time in his prison cell to reconsider his get-rich-quick scheme. We would all agree that Larry's investment plan was incredibly stupid because, in the end, he was severely punished and destitute. We would never do such a dumb thing as that. Would we? How often do we bankrupt our health by doing equally stupid things?

We take the time to maintain our cars, to change the oil, replace the filters, and check fluids every 3000 miles. We rotate tires, get tune-ups, and replace plugs whether or not our vehicle is under warranty. We take good care of our homes, too, or hire a cleaning lady to dust, mop, vacuum, and scrub. Every few months we polish the furniture, clean the carpet, scour the oven, and wash windows. We clean out the refrigerator and wax the floors. Why do we take the time and spend the money for all this work? Of course, we do it because we must. Our cars will break down and cost us more to repair or replace than if we had done the preventative maintenance. The brakes, tires, and hoses might fail and seriously injure someone. We maintain our homes because they look better when we take care of them. Having a clean, attractive home and car puts us at ease so that we feel good about ourselves and can feel superior to messy neighbors.

Do we treat our bodies as good? Most of us would rather eat worms than schedule a mammogram or a prostate exam. We wait until a toothache is driving us up the wall before we set foot in a dentist's office. Rather than see a doctor, we buy enough painkillers, laxatives, stool hardeners, fever medicines, indigestion soothers, and nasal decongestants to convince any alien that we are the sickest occupants of the galaxy. We act this way because the physician might poke us in some private place; or, worse, he might find something awful in one of those places. When we are really sick, we want a quick fix – a pill to make the pain go away, pare off 50 pounds overnight, or stop our craving for a cigarette. We want that fix yesterday, regardless of the fact that, for decades, we've ignored all preventative care. We'd never consider ignoring our cars and homes this way.

Does it make sense to take better care of our money than our bodies? Our bodies break down if we don't maintain them. Bypass surgery for a sticky heart valve can wreck our appointment book for months. Dirty lungs cost a bunch of money to fix, if they are repairable. We don't look so good after chemo or radiation treatment for a cancer we missed because we were too busy to have a physical. Nor will we play much tennis after we suffer a stroke because we ignored our sky-high blood pressure. Of course, we would agree that our bodies are as important as our vehicles; and we can't trade them in for a newer model, much as we would sometimes like to. We suggest that a better way to keep our engines running smoothly is to work on becoming wellthy.

Wellth results from investing in your body, your mind, and your spirit of self. Like amassing financial riches, you become wellthy by making frequent, small contributions to all these parts of you, not simply to your fiscal existence. The process is nothing like love at first sight or a bolt of lightning, for gathering wellth takes time, just as it does to grow your 401k or IRA accounts. Wellth investments earn interest that COMPOUNDS as your accounts grow, while DIVERSIFYING and BALANCING your wellth maximize your gains. Diversification is trying sardine soup and bungee jumping, or anything else you've always wanted to do. Your life is balanced when all the many sides of your diet, physical condition, personal, social and spiritual spheres are in synch with one another; or, to be more realistic, they are moving toward equilibrium. A balanced life, like a Buddhist state of enlightenment, is a process with no finish line. Beating yourself up with starvation diets or never taking time to do the things you love, be they drawing cartoons or crocheting collars for your boa constrictor, is way out of balance.

The 3 major components of wellth are comfortable eating, rewarding exercise, and personal growth. Each one takes time and effort to generate the ultimate dividend of a joyous, passionate, satisfying life, on most days, anyway. A bonus is that you secure wellth the same way you build wealth, in your STYLE, by defining and refining what you eat and how you exercise your mind and body, without orders or scolding from us. (What your mother says is another matter.) Fortunately, you have a smorgasbord of options from which to select a wellth portfolio that reflects your style. The first item to put on your plate is a description of your present health similar to the way you defined your current financial status. The following checklist is a guide to rating your health assets and liabilities.

____________________'s Health Investments Now

(Insert your name)

Be truthful if you can - no one is looking.

About food	Agree	Disagree
I'm more than 20 pounds overweight.	_____	_____
I eat a lot of junk food.	_____	_____
I don't like most vegetables.	_____	_____
I don't eat much fresh fruit.	_____	_____
Whole grains are for cows to eat.	_____	_____
I eat fast food because I'm so busy.	_____	_____
I'm a sugar/chocolate freak.	_____	_____
I love anchovies.	_____	_____
I go on food binges.	_____	_____
Sometimes I starve myself.	_____	_____

I'm on a diet most of the time. _____ _____

I eat when I'm depressed/stressed. _____ _____

I eat too much at parties. _____ _____

(Clue: Most people hate anchovies: this is a trick question.)

About exercise: (Circle those that describe you)

I sit most of the day.

Exercise is boring.

I don't have time to exercise.

I exercise like crazy on vacations.

I work out every day.

Exercise is useless for me.

I'm too tired to exercise.

I don't walk if I can ride.

At work, I use the elevators, not the stairs.

(Clue: Even triathletes take an occasional time out.)

About habits:

I drink more than 3 shots of alcohol a day.

(3 beers or glasses of wine or a 1 jigger cocktail)

I drink a lot on weekends.

I go on binges.

I drink when I am depressed/stressed.

I drink too much at parties.

I smoke cigarettes.

I smoke more when I'm depressed/stressed.

I use other addictive substances.

I do drugs when I'm depressed/stressed.

I don't take an annual physical exam.

I don't go to the dentist regularly.

I don't protect myself from AIDs or other venereal diseases.

About feelings:
I often feel depressed.
I'm not satisfied with my sex life.
I'm not satisfied with my job.
Life is hard and then you die.
Diamonds are a girl's best friend.
I seldom laugh out loud.
Not many funny things happen in my life.
I'd like to find the perfect high (cheap and no hangover).
It's hard for me to relax.
I don't have many friends.
I'm not close to my family.
(Clue: Who wouldn't want the perfect high? Read on.)

You probably noticed that the more statements you agree with, the less you have invested in your health. Not to worry: All these statements are about behaviors YOU control. No one forces double bacon-cheeseburgers or 6-packs of beer down your throat. You can choose not to smoke cigarettes or use dangerous drugs or risk a STD infection. You can flex your muscles even if you sit at a desk all day, you are able to eat wheat bread not cake, and you can find silly things to laugh about. Unlike monetary investments, choosing to be wellthy is utterly safe with few risks lurking in the background. This is a big plus because there ARE threats to your health you cannot change, such as your age, race, sex, past health history, and family health history. You can't help it if your blood relatives died from heart disease, obesity, or stroke. You aren't responsible for the diabetes, kidney disease, or cancer that runs in your family; but you can choose to act in ways that minimize these inherent risks.

You may be wondering how we can say that getting healthy isn't at all risky. People can go jogging and break a leg. Star athletes have been known to drop dead on the street and high school kids have heart attacks on the practice field. Like a profitable financial investment, it is highly probable that taking steps to improve our health will grant us a longer, more pleasant existence, though these steps don't guarantee that everyone will win all the time. We do know for certain that inactivity and overeating increase the risk of developing cancer by as much as 40% and they contribute substantially to practically all diseases, including depression. For instance, obese patients with heart disease die an average of 4 years earlier than patients of normal weight. Men who speed walk, jog, or play tennis every day live 8.7 years longer than their couch potato neighbors. Even moderate activity, such as golfing and walking, adds 5.8 years on average to your life expectancy. That's over 2000 more days to play catch with the grandkids, safari in Africa, and eat pizza in exchange for shaping up. Will you exercise your option on those bonus days?

Ambitious Annie's family history placed her at risk for early-onset diabetes, as well as heart disease. A physical exam revealed that she had a mildly elevated blood pressure and a 20- pound weight gain since her previous exam. Annie used to play soccer, now she coaches. She used to eat a healthy diet, now she's "too busy" to think about what she is eating. Feeling tired and weak, she finally dragged herself into her physician's office, where together they assessed her general health and set goals for the next 6 months. Her goals are to lose 20 pounds and reduce her blood pressure 20 points within a year. In the first 3 months, she's lost 5 pounds and lowered her pressure to 140 over 90. Annie now chicken steps her way to wellth by shunning fast food joints and packing her own lunch. When she goes out for a business meal, she replaces the steak and fries special with a chef's salad dressed in balsamic vinaigrette. She also walks a mile a day and can hardly wait to get out on the soccer field again in the spring.

A one-week goal of losing 5 pounds is not appropriate for anyone, nor is trying to run 5 miles a day if you've moved no faster than a two-toed sloth for the last 10 years. Just as investing small amounts of money over long periods of time makes us rich, one less cookie, one more flight of stairs climbed, one less extra helping at dinner, one more lap around the mall enriches our health. As pounds drop away, we are able to move more easily. When we walk or bike or bowl a little faster, we step up our metabolism and magnify our efforts, like compounding interest on our money. A big dividend is zapping the blues that attack us, especially when we step in front of a mirror.

Joining the 200 Club will increase your wellth at least as much as it boosts your financial portfolio. Eliminate 200 calories a day by eating a tad less, exercising a dab more, or both. You save this many calories by eating a cup of pasta instead of two cups and by walking 1 ½ miles in a half-hour. The following day, you might replace a piece of cake with a cup of low-fat yogurt, or lug 25 pounds of baby or potatoes in a backpack for half an hour. Either choice alone will earn your 200 for that day. Because 200 calories is such a miniscule amount, you probably won't miss 10 French fries or 20 potato chips. It's easy to squeeze in a brief half-hour of leaf raking, dancing, or other moderate activity every day. Better yet, make it a family 200-a-day- contest with prizes each month for all the winners. In 17 or 18 days, you'll have invested a pound off your butt or gut; AND you'll harvest the dividend of a sturdier heart.

To join the Club, you can track your 200 Club Points or Body Bucks in one of two ways. You can go to the Toy Store and buy play money which will be used for your Body Bucks. Make each bill equal to 100 calories. Please do not copy real currency on your copy machine as you may get a visit from the Treasury Department and then be led away in handcuffs. Prison food would not be a good way to lose weight. Your PLAY MONEY will go in an envelope labeled **WELLTH**. While your daily goal is to save 200 Body Bucks (calories) a day, add a Buck for every 100 you invest (each 100 calories saved over first 200) because we don't want you to freak when you fall short of your target. The second way to track your Body Bucks is by using a Pocket Check Register from any bank. Each time you save your daily calories, enter the date, mark "Calories Saved" in Payee area, and add as you would a deposit. Then balance the checkbook.

Of course, you can skip a day if you have to but you should then save double the next. Do not make this a habit. Struggling to eat 400 or 500 calories less per day is too difficult to maintain, something like saving a fourth of your salary, and you'll soon give up. On average, there will be 20 pounds less of you in one year when you set aside a trifling

200 calories every day. At this rate, you'll shed 3500 calories every 17.5 days or so, paring 72,000 fat ones in a year by eating a tiny bit less and exercising a tiny bit more. Don't fret about a pound more or less as your actual weight loss will vary from week to week.

We hear grumbles that you don't want to wait a whole year to slim down. "Can't I shed pounds faster?" Be reassured, you won't wait a year. When you dispense with 200 calories each and every day, you should see results on the scales in a month. The longer you belong to the 200 Club, the more you'll lose. In fact, one study found that the peak weight loss came 30 months after participants began a calorie-counting program. Heavies can take heart from findings that the more you weigh, the faster and the more pounds you'll lose. "But," you reply, "I've tried every diet known to humankind and I've failed again and again. Why should I join the Club?"

The good news is that investing in your health is completely different from dieting. The sole purpose of dieting is to lose weight. The purpose of eating for wellth is to gradually improve your body, without making drastic changes in what you eat. Don't think of it as dieting, since paring 200 calories a day isn't a gargantuan sacrifice. And, you can still eat to-die-for cheesecake and deep-dish pizza, once in a while. The principles of successful wealth building work even better for your WELLTH than they do for your money because:

1. Saving 200 calories a day pays far better dividends in a year than 200 cents a day.
2. Investing in your body pays off, no matter how old you are when you start.

3. You can lose your life savings in one night in Vegas. If the damage is not too severe, lungs, livers, and hearts usually can reverse the destruction caused by obesity, smoking, drinking, or drugs.
4. You need not wait 25 or 30 years to collect your wellth investments. With steady contributions, expect to see and feel the effects of compounding in 6 months.
5. Wellth dividends and interest aren't taxable at any age.
6. Having wellth may save a bundle of wealth in lost wages and medical bills. If you smoke a pack of cigarettes a day, quitting will net you $2500 a year.
7. There is no wellth inflation.
8. You can grow wellthy in the style of your choice.
9. When you are wellthy, you increase your chances of living long enough to spend your millions playing tennis, fly fishing, or counting your cash rather than lying in a hospital bed or a box.

To begin building wellth, forget about dieting and toss your diet books, all of them, because dieting is unnatural.

CHAPTER 3. DIETS AND OTHER UNNATURAL ACTS

Dieting, weighing yourself twice a day, reciting skinny mantras and pasting pig pictures on the door of the fridge guarantee frustration. How would you feel if you were told you couldn't take a shower or soak in the tub for the rest of your natural life? After a few days, wouldn't you do anything for a bath? Would you wait until the house was empty and leap into the shower, telling yourself, "I deserve it. I've been good. I'll give up showers tomorrow. My kids gave me this bath brush and I don't want to hurt their feelings." Try going without bathing for a week if you aren't convinced. Your mind will drive you straight to water, even if it's a teacup full.

Dieting is America's number one sport, far surpassing sleeping late and stealing paper clips, a sport in which at least half of us participate at some point in our lives; and 65 million of us are practicing at this moment. If we are female, 60 % of us play this dieting game all the time and most of us think about doing it for our entire earthly existence. (The second most popular sport is paying for dieting to the tune of 45 or 50 billion a year.) Some of us are so fond of it we start a diet every day. We gulp pills that promise to melt our fat, drink diet liquids laced with chemicals and preservatives, and buy anything labeled "lite" from plastic ice cream to reduced calorie radishes. Part of the fun is spending our life savings on food that looks yummy in the pictures and tastes like cotton balls. We get hypnotized, acupunctured, pummeled, and steamed to shed our fat. When these don't help, we join diet programs for the privilege of being abused by counselors so skinny they vanish when they turn sideways. These size 4 gurus of girth always know when you ate two corn chips yesterday, which is NOT ALLOWED. They are obsessed with weighing you so they can fiddle with the scales, making it appear that you've gained 10 pounds since leaving home an hour ago. "It's OK, dear," they murmur, "Fork over another $500 and we'll whip you into shape." They have plenty of job security knowing that 60% of adults and 25% of kids in the United States are overweight. Despite their threats and all the helpful aids, such as low calorie ham made from minced gopher ears or cattle feed ingeniously fashioned to resemble whipped cream, most of us would rather read tax manuals for the remainder of our lives than go on a diet for even one week. Why is dieting so unnatural to us? For several reasons, starting with the fact that most:

1. Diets are Deprivation. Invariably, diets require giving up foods you would give your first Rolls Royce for. They ignore the life-giving force of fudge-ripple ice cream or the restorative powers of blueberry pancakes slathered with butter and floating in syrup. They fail to understand that your stomach cannot grasp the meaning of just one French fry or that you would just as soon eat paper napkins as a baked potato with-

out sour cream, butter, and salt. We think of a diet as a temporary torture meant to peel off pounds quickly. It has to be quick because a life without fried onion rings isn't worth living. So, we tape our lips shut and emulate Cinderella, expecting the fairy godmother in charge of fat to transform us from slob to svelte at the stroke of midnight, or at least to the moment when we step on the scales again. Diets promise to melt our flab like butter on a steaming ear of corn and we greedily swallow this bit of hocus pocus.

Rita Rigorous decided she must lose 25 pounds to be a stunning maid-of-honor at her sister's wedding. Since she had only 2 months to prepare, she whittled her waistline with a vengeance, eating a scant 600 calories a day. She also got wrapped, massaged, and re-wrapped. It worked. Rita looked svelte and glamorous at the wedding and gratefully soaked up all the "oohs and ahs" that people heaped on her. Four months later, she was 10 pounds heavier and more discouraged than when she started.

Yes, diets do work whether they are pretty pink cans of diet water, diet dust in bright packages, grapefruit and vinegar diets, gerbil food diets, ham and egg diets. If your metabolism is speedier than a slug's, you'll lose weight quickly eating any low calorie, high carb, low carb, high fat, high protein or any kind of diet. Researchers at a major hospital in New York found that losing weight isn't the problem. Most of the people they examined dropped pounds like lead weights on a variety of diets, losing an average of 1½ to 2 pounds a week. But 50% of them fled the program before reaching their desired weights and immediately began to regain what they had struggled to lose. A scant 2% managed to keep the weight off for 5 years. Other studies show that 90% of dieters regain their weight within 2 years. Why is it so difficult to swap cookies for bean sprouts even when we are certain to lose weight if we do? A subtler factor than deprivation is at work and it is the second reason for diet failure:

2. Diets forbid DIVERSITY. Most of them allow only a very narrow range of foods, such as celery and carrot sticks or steak and cheese, with nothing to break the monotony. Since humans have been stealing eggs and eating everything from raw oysters to chocolate-covered roaches for several hundreds of thousands of years, it seems clear to us that we are programmed to consume a broad range of foods. Eating grains and meats, vegetables and fruits, nuts and milk is so natural to us after all these millennia that we cannot ignore our dietary heritage. Nor is there any need to ignore our heritage because a good diet, like a good investment, thrives on variety. Diets overlook something else and that is their third inherent problem. They aren't in balance.

3. BALANCE. Because they focus on eating, diets neglect a pivotal aspect of health: body balance. Body balance is the relationship between activity and eating, the equation of food consumed to exercise. A wellthy diet focuses not on eating, but on matching eating to action.

Puzzled Patrick, age 48, didn't exercise because he felt well and had lots of energy. A physical exam revealed that his health was excellent, except for one detail: he was getting older and his metabolism was slowing. "Why am I gaining weight," he asked, "when I'm eating no more than I did 20 years ago?"

Like Patrick, most of us maintain the same diet but exercise much less as we get older. This combination is guaranteed to expand our waistlines given that most of us need 100 calories or so less per day for each decade we live after age 25. If he ate 3500 calories a day when he was 28, Patrick should take in 3300 calories now, less another 200 because he is sedentary. By age 40, people who get no exercise beyond getting in and out of their cars tend to wrap a pound of fat a year around their bodies. You may weigh the same as before, but now it is fat, not muscle. Bone loss in sedentary, post-menopausal women magnifies this effect, making exercise critical to maintaining their body balance as they age. Patrick joined the 200 Club and began paring his lard by eating less fried chicken and more chard and collards without bacon, healthy greens he liked because they reminded him of home. He earned another 200 body bucks doing what he got a kick out of, training his quarter horse and playing sand volleyball. He's proud of himself for controlling his weight, a well-deserved pride that motivates him to stay in the 200 Club. The last and most powerful reason of all for why diets fail is that -

4. Diets belong to Strangers. People with the physiques of a praying mantis invent diets, the ones who appear to have gained slightly more than their birth weights and whose vision of paradise is a 20-foot stack of raw broccoli. They demand that we spread bran, not butter, on our bread, eat sprouts not sukiyaki, and learn to love anything raw. They deny us that uplifting glass of wine before dinner, insisting we risk drowning while chug-a-lugging enough water to flush Seattle straight into the Pacific. They sentence us to a life without

cheese fries and peanut butter and jelly sandwiches, a regime as alien to us as mealy worms and alligator eyes.

Someone else's diet, no matter how good for us it is, simply will not work when it clashes with our style. We balk when we are forced to give up foods as comfortable as old jeans. A successful diet, meaning one we will stick to for more than 2 hours, is one we choose for ourselves. Once we decide what we will eat and when we will eat it, we'll stay with the program. Diets fail not because they don't work but because they aren't us.

Did you know that your menu is far older than you are? It's composed of your mother's diet, your father's favorite foods, and the good stuff your aunts and cousins and nieces brought to family celebrations. Their menus, in turn, catch the flavors of their predecessors from eons before. What you like to eat is infused with half-remembered images of the atmosphere in which your family cooked. It's spiced by the memory of the people with whom you shared your meals and the places where you dined. This is why an aroma can evoke a rush of nostalgia for mom's or nana's apple cobbler or kugel or coffee cake. Vivid pictures of the bread grandma baked flash across the memory screen in our brains, or you catch a glimpse of the strawberry shortcake she made with from-scratch biscuits and freshly whipped cream. More images pop up: pictures of the long table where you ate, papa at one end carving the chicken, mama calling you to pass your plate to her while your brother pinches you, hoping you'll drop it. Next time you talk about food, do you picture where and with whom you ate it? Your diet is seasoned with your cultural traditions, such as the pot of marinara sauce simmering on the back burner or the brown bread steaming in the oven. The family's religious rituals of a boisterous brunch after mass or cake and cherry phosphates at the close of the Sabbath round out your personal menu. It's a diet both intimate and complex; diet strangers know nothing about you. You are expected to abandon your past and present traditions and dine with people you never met. The problem is that, no matter how much you try, you can't be someone else. Your diet is like an anchor, holding you in place.

Fad diets work for a while, then fail. Why? Picture yourself as a high-powered speedboat tethered to a massive iron anchor, scrapping along the sea bottom. You gun your engine and race through the waves, trailing a wake of churning water behind. It's a glorious ride until the line goes taut. It yanks you backward with a hull-splitting jolt. You stop dead. The engine conks out. The boat starts to sink with you in it. There is no way you can go forward until you raise the anchor, link by link, out of the water.

You can't eat wellthy on your mother's diet, your friend's, your spouse's diet, or diets you study in books. The only possible way you will ever eat wellthy is to follow your own personal menu, a menu reflecting your history and traditions and cravings. To hoist your anchor, take the time to **DEFINE** your present diet. You can't fix something until you know what is broken. Think about what you eat at home and what you order at a restaurant. Remember your must-have to-die-for foods (these are the things that, once eaten, you can't live without), the dishes that you grew up with, the ones you hold dear.

Dr. S's are Krispy Kreme Donuts, Friendly's Ice Cream, and Renee's cheesecake. Dr. P's are steamed mussels fresh from the ocean and maple syrup mousse made with real whipped cream. Struggling to give them up is useless for they define your diet, foods worth saving up enough body bucks to splurge on.

Compulsive Cathy is a 37-year-old computer systems engineer and single mom. She kept the baby and 50 extra pounds after she delivered her second child and her husband walked out. Bothered by swollen ankles and chest pains, she read diet books and joined weight-loss programs. They did nothing for her. Cathy defined her menu, hour by hour, for 2 weeks on computer spreadsheets (we recommend smart phone apps) that had cells for calorie counts, percentages of hydrogenated and saturated fats, both kinds of cholesterol, sodium, carbohydrates, fiber, protein, vitamins, calcium, and iron. Her "can't live without foods" were crunchy ones, like potato chips, and ones she didn't have to cook. Listing the details of her menu reflected her style and made her feel in control.

Jolly Jim, an overweight diabetic man in his early fifties, had a much different style. Because he traveled constantly on business, he knew his favorite restaurants better than his own kitchen. Jim defined his diet one night as he grazed on the entire basket of crusty French bread and creamy butter, waiting for the chef to grill his T-bone medium rare, crisp the fries, and dish up the salad before dessert of ba-ba rum cake covered with whipped cream. That fabulous bread was a keeper, he thought, a "will-not-do-without food." Maybe he could give up the cake, but never the bread. He felt confident that he could handle his choices. By defining their diets in their individual styles, Cathy and Jim could start taking small steps to make their menus work for them without dragging them backward.

Now, it's your turn to define your dietary self, as you are now.

______________________________'s DIET NOW

Your name here

What I ate in the past 3 days:

____

____

____

____

____

____

____

My Can't Do Without Foods are:

____

____

____

____

Give yourself a hug. You have taken the first step in controlling your Menu instead of letting it control you. Your next step is to steer around an illness that plagues most of us at some point in our lives, an illness we call Diet Dis-ease.

CHAPTER 4.
DIET DIS-EASE

Dis-ease. Heart disease. Lung disease. Kidney disease. The word describes the pain and malaise we feel when we are sick. We dread serious diseases; we fear the possibility even of confronting them. We gulp handfuls of Vitamin C to avoid catching colds and beg for bottles of antibiotics to squelch the ones that catch us. We want to be comfortable in our skins, at ease with our bodies. We want to be at ease with food, too; but many of us are anything but. We suffer from diet dis-ease.

Diet dis-ease is punishing ourselves by forgoing the foods that define us: the fluffy biscuits draped with cream gravy, greasy tacos, and lacy crullers. We are too heavy and must suffer for it. When no one is looking, we tiptoe to the freezer and inhale a quart of butter pecan ice cream in one sitting. Immediately, we hate ourselves and swear to ingest nothing but celery and water until we turn into dust. We aren't even at ease when we're not hungry; so we nosh, gobbling everything in sight, centerpiece included. Now, we have the "guilties" and must graze on bacon rinds for solace. "It's a shame to waste food. I can't offend my hostess. I'll take just one itsy bite." There is no end to our excuses. The most severe food disease is bingeing followed by induced vomiting or purging with laxatives to expel the dreadful stuff we were forced to eat. None of these behaviors are about feeling hungry. They mirror our scrambled emotions, not the pleasure of eating. They apply every bit as much to the excessive use of alcohol, drugs, and cigarettes as they do to food. So, how do we know when we're truly hungry, rather than mad or sad or just plain bored? Don't blame the pangs and growls of your stomach; blame your brain.

Your tummy may rumble, gurgle, burble, and chirp; but it's not the boss. An eating center, in the hypothalamus, deep in the middle of your brain, runs the show. It sends messages via the blood stream to your stomach telling it when to dish up the food. This restaurant in your head works in tandem with an adjacent parking lot, called the satiety center. When your meal has filled all the parking spaces, the satiety center tells your stomach it is full and tells you to stop eating.

This is a fine system, as without it we either would eat until we exploded or refuse food while we starved to death. These eating and stop eating centers are interconnected with brain mechanisms regulating body temperature, explaining why we may feel cold when we're hungry and sweat when we eat. Two-way connections also link our eating centers to systems that manage our feelings of pleasure, fear, anger, and fatigue. This intricate network influences messages from our "eat, don't eat" centers, making it easy for us to confuse emotions with hunger. When you are scared out of your wits, do you eat everything that doesn't run or do you practically gag at the thought of food? Does either happen when you are red in the face angry or so sad you'd like the whole box of macaroni and cheese?

Messages from our brain café telling us to begin eating take 20 to 30 minutes to reach our stomachs. This delay may explain why some people get crabby or have splitting headaches when they are hungry. Our "don't eat" signals are equally pokey, sometimes so slow our stomachs don't know the parking lot is full and continue to demand food. Eating a meal in less than ½ hour may be so fast that we eat more than we need or want because our stomach didn't get the message. This is particularly true when we skip breakfast or cram calories at night, and then do penance until we are hungry enough to eat anything that doesn't talk back. Become the maitre d' of your brain café by eating slowly for at least half an hour; and no, you don't have to chew each bite 30 times. If you think dining for 30 minutes is easy, time yourself at your next meal. Like filling up at the gas station, most of us stuff and run when we could spend more time savoring each bite of our dinner without becoming a giant kielbasa sausage.

Another reason for eating when we aren't hungry is that, like combustion engines and gasoline, celebrations and food go together. Can you imagine a wedding reception without a towering rosette-strewn cake? Or a kid's birthday party with no tri-color ice cream? A family Thanksgiving dinner devoid of a massive turkey with all the trimmings? What would Easter, Passover, Christmas, or Hanukkah be with nothing to eat? For that matter, imagine if you can, a tailgate party or family reunion without food. We soon learn that eating is for feel-good times, times we spend with other people, times when boredom and loneliness vanish.

Before Lent and after Sabbath or Ramadan, we eat. We eat on dates, go on picnics in the park, pass dishes at pot-luck suppers, munch tidbits at cocktail parties, office parties, school parties, all parties. Food merchants in our cities hold food fests, the sole purpose of which is to encourage us to gobble their wares. Parents reward their children with yet more food: "If you clean your plate, you may have a cookie." We fight with food, throw pies in faces, even eat to honor our dead. Even at a wake, we commiserate and comfort each other over chicken casseroles and cherry pies.

Gregarious Gloria grew up in a robust family whose social life revolved around eating. "People were always coming and going at our house," she said, "and eating. When we talked about anything: money, family, school, it was always at the kitchen table piled with food. It seems like it was yesterday," she added, "that people came over for birthdays and weddings, carrying platters heaped with red cabbage and sausages, goulash and dumplings, and oh, that wonderful poppy-seed cake they baked."

Gloria has a demanding full-time job in the family business but she still cooks constantly for dinner parties, graduations, and baby showers. "I like to be around people," she declared with a smile, "surrounded by love, laughing, and lots of good things to eat." Other than a few extra pounds and bouts of heartburn, Gloria's health is very good, in part because she balances her eating with rushing about to shop for food, cook, and clean up. Then, she starts all over again the next week. Her passion for pleasing people and receiving their warmth in return enhances the balance in her life.

Not all of us manage Gloria's equilibrium. When a boyfriend dumps us, an entire chocolate chip cheesecake offers us immense solace, while half a pound of bonbons works wonders after a fight with our spouse. We destroy a deep-dish pizza when the boss has a fit and demolish a full slab of ribs if we don't get that raise. We soothe our children's pain with food, too, when we tell our children, "I'm sorry that shot hurt; let's go for ice cream." It's no wonder we grow fat when food becomes our parent, lover, chaplain, and mentor. The next time you reach for a cupcake, ask yourself, "Am I hungry or do I need a hug?" If you're hungry, eat! If you want a friendly squeeze, ask someone for a bear hug. Wrap your arms around yourself if no one is available, as strangers may take a dim view of your request.

Don't deny your emotions because they are genuine, though they may be badly misplaced. Is Rocky Road ice cream really your best friend or your security blanket? Is it easier to gobble the Danish than to deal with your feelings? Figure out when you are tired and reach for a cup of tea, not the fudge cake. Popping Oreos or downing another cocktail won't erase our emotions, only our attitudes can do that. The next time you are stressed out, stop crunching the corn chips and indulge in a good cry. Walk around the block as fast as you can. Telephone a friend. Scribble down your feelings, letting them shout and sob on paper. When you're ready, inhale slowly, exhale more slowly, and ask yourself, "Am I still hungry? Will I delight in the delicious taste of every bite I take? Will I feel at ease when I'm finished eating?" If so, it's time for your snack. Practicing these chicken steps probably won't make us slim but they may help us recognize what triggers us to eat too much. We can then define our menu sufficiently to know what we can scratch and what are our "to-die-for" dishes.

For starters, DEFINE your triggers. Let's look at our triggers to eating when we aren't really hungry. This compulsive kind of eating usually involves foods high in fats and/or sugars, such as cupcakes and pies, French fries and cheeseburgers, donuts and chips. All of us, (except food saints and we don't know any), are susceptible to Frito attacks and cheesecake ambushes. Some of us are secret nibblers who eat gustily when we are alone but starve ourselves when someone is looking. Others among us devour the canapes at parties by the fistfuls. Often, we nosh when we are feeling sad or angry or bored, but not all of us do. All-purpose eaters are flexible: they eat in the lunch room at work, at the grocery store (where some of us sneak furtive bites of stolen goodies), or when the kids won't clean their plates and it's a shame to pitch them. Sometimes, we eat because we're supposed to. If you are eating lunch because it's time for lunch, put down your fork. Are you chowing down because you're hungry? Because the food smells so good? Because it's parked in front of you begging to be devoured, because you paid for it and you're going to get your money's worth? Because it's free? If you aren't hungry, don't eat it. If you're a little hungry, nibble on your bagel and feed the dog the rest. This checklist may help you discover your personal triggers to food attacks, although you may already know them all too well.

I eat when I'm feeling: (Circle those that apply to you)

Stressed
Angry
Bored
Depressed
Guilty
Excited
Frustrated
Lonely
Scared
Tired
Very happy
Other ________________________________

I eat when I'm:

At parties
At grocery stores
In malls
Watching TV
At bedtime
At work
On weekends
My usual mealtimes
Reading at my computer
Other places where I eat ____________________

The times when I'm most likely to over eat are:

Early mornings
Midmornings
Early afternoons
Late afternoons
Early evenings
Late at night

Compulsive Cathy's spreadsheets startled her. Here's a summary of one of her pages: 7:00 A.M. drive to daycare and work; bagels and coffee in the van; 10:00 A.M. work break, diet soda; 1:00 P.M. lunch at desk, diet soda; 6:00 P.M. drive home from work, pick up kids, stop for sausage pizza and pop with the kids; 8:30 P.M. get kids to bed, do work from office, ½ box of caramels; 11:00 P.M. in bed with bag of chips and dip.

Cathy's emotions overwhelmed her at night when she was tired and stressed by the responsibilities of her job and being a good mother. After reviewing her list, she realized that, when the kids were asleep and the ticking of the clock was the only noise in the house, she struggled to fill the emptiness inside her with food.

As you might expect, Jolly Jim's checklist was quite different from Cathy's. Wondering why he couldn't lose weight when he wasn't eating all that much, he dictated a few notes on his pocket recorder. Here's what he learned on a typical weekday: 7:00 A.M. bacon and eggs, toast and hash browns at a restaurant; 8:00 A.M. candy bar driving to meet a customer; 10:00 A.M. birthday cake and coffee with customer;

12:00 noon, double cheeseburger, fries, and soda at a fast food place; 3:00 P.M. cheese and crackers; 6:30 P.M. chips and soda from the motel room mini fridge; 7:30 P.M. surf and turf dinner out with a customer; 10:00 P.M. cheese pretzels and candy from the mini fridge. It was evident to him that he ate to quell the loneliness of being on the road, feelings exacerbated by the ready availability of food he didn't have to lift a finger to cook. Once Cathy and Jim understood why they ate too much, they could get comfortable with eating without overindulging when they were lonely or stressed. They were ready to refine their menus and be comfortable with the component of wellth that we call "food-ease."

CHAPTER 5.
FOOD-EASE

Dr. S. is passionate about popcorn. He eats it every night. He adores its crunch; he treasures its clean, crisp taste. The microwave version is so convenient, he used to buy it by the case until he read the label. Because he devoured the entire package, his munchies were costing him 360 calories and 32 grams of fat every night. He sampled another brand. It weighed in at 345 calories and 10.5 grams of fat. A third product yielded 240 calories and 5 grams of fat. It tasted fine. Over the next 2 weeks, he pared his portion to half the bag, one cup at a time, for a grand total of 120 calories, 2.5 grams of fat, and half the salt of the first 2 products. By refining his menu in chicken steps, he saved 240 calories and nearly 30 grams of fat without craving more. Dr. S. had discovered food-ease.

Food-ease (not foodies!) is eating when we are hungry and enjoying every bite. It engages all our senses: the mellow aroma of freshly-baked bread, the eye-catching glamour of precisely-arranged sushi or cobb salad, the sizzle of chicken on the grill, the velvety mouth feel of frozen yogurt, and, of course, the tangy-sweet taste of ripe, straight from-the-garden tomatoes. We are at ease with food when we delight in eating, not to bury our feelings or please our moms, but for its own sake. Taking extravagant pleasure in eating is not a crime; it is feeling alive and good about yourself. Since cold-turkey diet restrictions have inherent problems, we recommend making small adjustments in your menu to reduce your calories and expand your choices. While you're at it, refine the family's menu, too. Hang on to your Haagen-Dazs and play the incredible Shrinking Scoop game. If you normally dish out 3 heaping scoops, try serving 2 1/2 scoops until you are satisfied with the smaller portion. Then try dishing up 2 scoops, then 1 ½, till you can nosh for a half hour on just one scoop. After a few weeks, your tummy will feel full and you will pocket 250 body bucks each time you reduce the scoop by ½ cup. Your parents may have used this sneaky trick to wean you from your precious security blanket by stealthily snipping away at your beloved rag until it was 2 inches square and you forgot about it. Scoop less than a cup if you like, but don't give up all ice cream if it's one of your can't-live-without foods. Treat all your goodies equally: cut 1 ½ pieces of chocolate cake if you customarily eat 2, 4 fistfuls of potato chips instead of 5, 3 slices of pepperoni pizza in place of 4. If arithmetic isn't your forte, eyeball your normal portions and shrink them a wee bit, one at a time. The idea is to savor, in small bites, the portions you take without fretting that you may have taken 2¼ servings instead of 2. As you whittle away at your food, you will reach "critical mass." When 2 ¼ cups makes you happy and 2 cups makes you want to go back for seconds, you've reached your critical mass (CM). Enjoy your

2 ¼ cups and never eat less. Move on to other foods and discover their CM. Body bucks add up quickly with chicken step refinements like these in your menu.

If the kids think cutting calories is as exciting as reading James Joyce, do a sleight of hand trick practiced by a billion Chinese. Dig out your wok or the largest frying pan you own, swipe it with oil and heat it till it begs for mercy. Meanwhile, cut in small pieces all the fresh veggies you can find: green beans, onions, red peppers, carrots, summer squash, celery, mushrooms, or anything else from the depths of your fridge and toss them into the wok. Stir for a minute or 2, and then sear a cup of thinly sliced raw chicken or steak for another couple of minutes. Splash with soy sauce, sesame oil, black bean curd, Thai chili sauce, or whatever seasonings you prefer, mix in a little cooked pasta, and dish it up. This pretty potpourri is pretty low in calories and fat but bursts with flavor and diverse textures.

For diners who insist on the separation of chard and steak, marinate thinly sliced beef or chicken in your choice of seasonings, roll the pieces in sesame or flax seeds, and skewer them. Grill briefly and dunk in the marinade after you broil it. Another trick is to slip soybean crumbles that masquerade as cooked hamburger into pasta sauce, tacos, or lasagna for a veggie treat that acts like meat. Add a bit of arrowroot or cornstarch to gravies to get the glossy look and velvety texture perfected by Oriental cooks. Try simmering veggies, even less than gorgeous ones, in water or tomato juice seasoned with bay leaf, wine, and perhaps a carcass leftover from the roast chicken, until you reduce the volume by half. Strain out the solids, skim the fat, and you have a low-cal broth suited to every dish. And, as grandma can tell you, chicken soup is good for everything that ails you.

Scaloppini offers another way to stretch calories like a giant rubber band. Your family will assume they are getting lots of them when what you've done is to spread a dietician's serving of meat across their entire plate. Buy cutlets, or slice at home skinny layers of turkey breast, chicken, veal, or lean pork. Beat them fiercely with a wooden mallet until they double in circumference. Then abuse them some more. Sauté them briefly, deglaze the pan with wine or tomato juice, and sprinkle with grated Parmesan to create a classic parmesan crusting. When you squirt it with lemon juice, it's a wiener schnitzel. Both dishes contain tons of flavor and not nearly as many calories as their taste suggests. If you're a cook, play with your favorite recipes to reduce the ingredients you want to banish without sacrificing flavor. Using no-fat mayonnaise in your potato salad eliminates 66% of the calories along with all that fat, while layering fruit or angel food cake with low-fat chocolate-raspberry or key lime yogurt creates a delicious and fat free parfait or tiramisu.

You may be wondering, how much is a serving? Your version might be a 1-pound T-bone or 3 cups of pasta swimming in meat sauce, topped off with a double dip chocolate cone. Alas, the dieticians have no sense of humor. To them, a serving of meat is the size of a deck of cards, meaning 3-4 ounces. It's one slice of bread or a scant cup of naked pasta. Half a cup of sauce is a second serving; a mere ½ cup of ice cream is a third. We define a serving as a little less than you are currently eating.

It's easy to be misled by the heaping platefuls dished up in restaurants that offer gargantuan portions to keep the customers coming back. Perhaps influenced by the "all you can eat" places, most of us believe we eat far less than we do and definitely more than what the standard food pyramid means by a serving. In a recent test, even registered dieticians grossly underestimated the calories in a typical restaurant offering of a grilled chicken Caesar salad. This dish contained 660 calories and 46 grams of fat, not the low counts you might expect in a salad. To understand quality rather than volume, dine at a good French or Japanese place, although you may wonder where all the food went. Decide if you want to experience perfection in taste, aroma and eye appeal, or shovel it in like a horse in a feedbag. The choice is yours. When you absolutely must have quantity, munch exploding food, such as lettuce and raw spinach (1 serving = 3 cups). Keep a bowl of fresh blueberries (a serving = 1 cup), strawberries, kiwis, or radishes on hand in place of cheese and crackers. Present a bowl of puffed anything: rice, oats, corn, pigeon, scattered with fresh berries for breakfast or as an anytime treat. Think up your own exploded treats (celery and popcorn) to diversify your menu.

On his next visit to the bread bistro, Jolly Jim asked his server to bring 4 slices, not the usual 8 slices of bread filling his basket. Instead of wolfing down the entire basketful, he nibbled at the slices leisurely. Grazing at half speed left him satisfied with 280 calories in place of 560 calories and smug that he saved more than his 200 calories by refining, not denying, his main, must-have menu item. Since Compulsive Cathy wasn't about to give up her bedtime crunchies, she shopped on the Internet for alternatives to potato chips that, at 10 calories a chip, 60% of them from fat, were not acceptable. She found veggie chips at 9 calories, ½ from fat, but this substitute didn't offer any real savings. One site she visited had a better idea. On some weekends, she and the kids microwaved piles of thinly sliced sweet potatoes, carrots, parsnips, and corn tortillas, lightly sprayed with canola oil and sprinkled with onion powder or cumin. They saved half the calories, 90% of the fat and salt, and 66% of the price of the store-bought chips. Finally, Cathy could curl up in bed with a snack that earned her body bucks. And the kids liked them, too. We won't lecture you about what you should or should not eat, as each of us must create our own refinements. We shall toss out tidbits for you to test, such as "Go Gaelic."

The next time you come home from work tired and hungry enough to eat a horse, do as the French do: leisurely nibble an hors d'oeuvre (pronounced "or der-urve," rhyming with nerve). These pre-dinner treats (antipasti to Italians) can be 2 servings of any food you like: an ounce of your favorite cheese with ½ cup of apple slices, a cup of steaming rigatoni with ½ cup of marinara sauce and a sprinkling of parmesan cheese; a latke with ½ cup of unsweetened apple sauce, a cup of borscht dolloped with plain yogurt; or a slice of toasted Italian bread rubbed with garlic in a cup of steaming minestrone. Pretend it's your life raft and push it around for a while like the kids do.

Soups, such as meatless matzo ball, low-fat split pea, or vichyssoise, are also satisfying hors d'oeuvres. Half a toasted bagel with ¼ cup of low-fat cream cheese is fine, too; and you can draw faces in the cheese. We can hear our mothers scolding in the background: "Don't snack before dinner. You'll spoil your appetite. You won't have room for your fried chicken."

Don't listen! You intend to "spoil" your appetite by giving your brain clock time to cancel that growling, empty stomach feeling while you relax. If you feel full half an hour after munching your granola bar, so much the better. Stop eating and think about how good you feel. Next, do as Europeans do: linger at the table for ½ hour with a glass of red wine or grape juice. In a few minutes, munch a hefty green salad sprinkled with olive oil and balsamic vinegar, or sip your soup if your hors d'oeuvre was a pear wrapped in proscuitto. Follow the salad with a cup of mashed potatoes creamed with buttermilk, a serving of white and brown rice risotto, or polenta (grits in the south) with a grating of Romano cheese. We guarantee you will feel as stuffed as a holiday turkey within an hour after you first sat down.

Nibbling works best if you prepare your canapés ahead of time, let the kids help prepare and eat the delectable goodies, and when you don't nosh while standing at the kitchen sink. Sit down and contemplate how pretty the food looks, not your list of chores or your fickle boss. Because they treasure good food for its own sake, the French cannot imagine dining in less than 2 or 3 hours. Take your time to chat with your family about friendly things (let the kids up when they ask to be excused for the 10th time) and concentrate only on tasting your meal, bite by bite. Forget the evening news for ½ hour and don't think of reading a book, even if you're eating solo. Do light a candle and play your favorite music. If your cooking is a disaster, play Wagner. Are you afraid you'll gobble everything in sight? If so, try lingering 15 minutes over a bruchetta of whole wheat toast spread with roasted red peppers and sprinkled with olive oil and grated cheese. Sip a drink of your choice and remember a funny thing that happened today. If you're still grabbing after 15 minutes, push your chair back and find other ways to refine your diet. For more nibble hints, check out the section on 25 more ways to foodease at the end of the book.

At first, you may feel anxious that you are wasting time, that you should be doing the laundry or yelling at the kids to do their homework, or reading that inane report from your office. We gulp our food without noticing how good it tastes and smells so that we can finish in 10 minutes. What for? To watch TV? Drive the kids somewhere? Do the dishes? Do our expense reports? Our lives depend on what we eat, yet we treat our meals like dirt to be swept out of sight as quickly as possible.

Have more fun with your food by practicing eating, Spanish style. Each evening they flock to bars, not to drink but to chat with their friends and nosh tapas, such as small snacks of fish, olives, veggies, and meats, served with a glass of sherry to be sipped till they get kicked out at closing time. For several thousand years, the Chinese have been nibbling without guilt on dainty dumplings filled with veggies or meat, called dim sum. Perhaps they know a thing or two about foodease. Order these delicacies at a restaurant or fix your own by bundling minced chicken, shrimp, and veggies in won ton wrappers. Steam them over simmering water and dip in the sauces of your choice.

"Get real!" some of us are muttering. "My husband is a meat and potato man and the kids are dessert-a-holics. They'll run screaming out the door when I bring out the antipasto. Besides, aren't Spanish tapas, Greek dolmades, or antipasti too oily to be good for you?"

The Mediterranean diet is based on olive oil that is very low in saturated fat. Italians eat far more veggies than we, some of which they prepare for hours, like beans and cardoon, a big thistle to us. Remember that they had the good sense to kidnap tomatoes and raise them as their own, the South American native that, at the time, was thought to be poisonous. Mediterranean people consume a little meat and a bit of wine, but usually reserve desserts for very special occasions. They toss a little sauce with their pasta, not the other way around. Maybe we should take a cue from them, as their incidence of heart disease and cancer is considerably less than ours.

Your family might delight in tapas when you announce that dinner is served on the patio table or rec room floor. Refine their meal in chicken steps, such as filling half their plates with salad in lieu of French fries and dinner rolls. Make pretty food, such as sliced oranges on baby greens, scattered with green grapes and shredded coconut. Decorate fresh pineapple slices with radish eyes, a carrot nose, red pepper mouth and shredded lettuce hair. Or make a little person with a cherry tomato head, celery stick limbs and lettuce clothes. Announce chicken for dinner and pass tofu fingers with low-cal salad dressing for dipping. Bite-size chunks of veggie wieners on toothpicks are good, too, since kids go for anything they can eat with their fingers. Spouses may take more persuasion. If you change gradually, by chicken steps, they will hardly notice as they slowly become wellthy.

For them, try low-fat frozen yogurt if you usually eat chocolate ice cream when you're watching TV together. Switch from baked potatoes with sour cream and butter to oven baked wedges lightly sprayed with olive oil and dashed with grated asiago cheese and garlic powder. Offer half the customary volume of bread spread with apple butter or hot pepper jelly for heat lovers. Present sliced peaches alongside the dobles torte, or make a fruit cobbler topped with granola mix. Whip up a chocolate mousse parfait using a mix and skim milk, then layer it with low-fat white chocolate yogurt and dollops of low-fat whipped topping. Top your masterpiece with berries or chocolate sprinkles.

About now, some of you are scoffing that making tiny tidbits and funny faces is wonderful if you love to cook, can afford to stay at home to do it, and have a maid to clean up after you. "I work long hours, travel for my job, chauffeur the kids, and look after my elderly mother. I DON'T COOK." When you would rather move in with your mother-in-law than cook, improvise your refinements. Order noshes on the Internet; or pick up noshes from your grocer's deli, a favorite restaurant, or specialty store if they don't deliver. Use a shopping service to collect your munchies or maybe entire meals while you collect the kids. Get together with a group of friends once a month to prepare tapas and dim sum for everyone's table and freezer. When you must eat and run, treat your offspring to a tailgate picnic antipasto in lieu of a fast food joint. Occasionally, let them prepare a meal to your specifications. If they want to avoid starvation, they will oblige, and maybe have fun doing it. And bear in mind that you're refining so that you CAN occasionally dive into the pepperoni pizza, chocolate truffles, or any of your to-die-for treats. Read on to discover more ways to refine yourself right into foodease.

CHAPTER 6.
GET REFINED

Macaroni and cheese, bacon and eggs, sausage gravy, and our other favorite foods feel rich and creamy in our mouths. Meat loaf with gravy, BBQ ribs, and pasta Alfredo glide over our tongues. Chocolate cream pie and strawberry cheesecake caress our palates. We cherish these foods for their "mouth feel." They relax us but they make us fat. By all means, relish your favorite fried chicken, enchiladas, or triple chocolate cake, but only in smaller portions. And search for ways to clone the satiny mouth sensation of your cozy foods.

Buttermilk is a creamy, satisfying substitute for mayonnaise salad dressings. You may object, "Buttermilk? It tastes awful. It's fattening." A bit of buttermilk feels like sour cream in cole slaw and on mashed potatoes. Add a little sugar and you will insist it is cream in cream pies. It contains no butter; in fact, it has half the fat of 2% milk. Since it probably won't work in crème brulle, prepare your version with fake eggs and lighter cream to dispense with over half the calories and 75% of the fat in the original. Or try sabayon using fake eggs and confectioner's sugar. This custard sauce is wonderful over everything from fresh fruit to old sneakers. Another fat-skimming trick is to make a smooth glossy gravy with broth or wine, after you banish the fat from the pan juices. As we mentioned, tofu, that rubbery-looking stuff made from soybeans, is a good stand-in for part of the meat in your stir fry, stews, and chilies. You won't miss the fat because tofu is smooth on the tongue and filling in the tummy despite being low in fat and high in protein. If you suffer from extreme tofu fear, use other reduced-fat products. Yogurt ice cream offers good mouth feel, as does low-fat cream cheese on your bagel and reduced-fat margarine on your veggies. Greek yogurt is high in protein and makes great dips. Make yogurt "cheese" by straining plain yogurt overnight in the frig using a sieve lined with cheesecloth. The water drains away, leaving the creamy solids to use in salad dressings and on vegetables. Or make a dip called laboneh by stirring in sesame seeds, savory, cumin, and a bit of olive oil into the drained yogurt. Served with toasted pita bread triangles, fresh radishes, and olives, this is a classic Israeli mezze, or appetizer.

Be wary of products labeled "low-fat, healthy, or diet." Maybe they are, maybe they aren't, and maybe the difference is so slight it makes no difference. For example, one popular brand of reduced-fat peanut butter has only 5 fewer grams of fat and 10 fewer calories than the regular version. Is this what you're looking for in a low-fat product? A brand name diet vanilla ice cream product does have less fat (2.5 vs 8 grams) but more calories (170 versus 140) than its regular vanilla counterpart. A "healthy" soup brand registers 10 more calories and ½ gram more fat than the manufacturer's regular vegetable soup, perhaps proving once again that we gorge on the advertising, rather than digesting the list of ingredients. Another trap to be weary of is that "white" meat is always better for you than the "red" stuff. You're better off eating lean ground sirloin containing 4 grams of fat and 130 calories per 3-ounce serving than a popular brand of ground turkey stuffed with 17 grams of fat and 230 calories. To lower both counts, choose skinless turkey breast. Lean beef is good for dinner, too. Check the fat content to see just how lean it really is.

Eating whole grains and beans provide interesting textures enriched with a fiber bonus. If dining on fiber sounds to you like eating hay, sample creamy risotto made with ½ brown and ½ basmati rice. Gradually add boiling broth as you stir and continue stirring until all the liquid is absorbed (tiring but worth the effort). If you hate to steam over a hot range, order it at a restaurant. Other choices include the weird-sounding grains called couscous (pronounced "coos-coos") and quinoa ("keen-wha"), both high-protein South American exports, and soba, a buckwheat noodle from Japan. While you are experimenting and refining, try buckwheat flour blinis and pancakes laced with a bit of wheat germ or whole wheat buds. Concoct bean smoothies like humus, a spread which is made from chick peas (garbanzos) ground with sesame seeds and herbs. Ground garbanzo patties, called falafel, are a popular Middle Eastern snack that you can make from scratch garnished with tomatoes, shredded lettuce, and onions. If dried beans render you socially unacceptable, eat these treats ½ cup at a time for a pleasant veggie break. They will reward you by quickly canceling the messages from your brain urging you to gorge yourself.

It's easy to be confused by the suggestions of experts who may or may not agree with one another. A new miracle food seems to crop up every month or two, followed by the latest forbidden food that was in vogue yesterday. To agitate us further, these two often change places. Just when we think we know a good choice from a bad one, the "experts" reverse their opinions. We should use My Plate (this used to be the Food Pyramid) as a guide, not our master. A medley of raw or steamed vegetables can be both filling and delicious. Think broccoli, carrots, spinach, and chard seasoned with rosemary, thyme, and oregano. This tasty dish provides variety and heaps of antioxidants. When you've had enough leaves, gnaw on a fresh peach or plum.

Let's go fishing. Some Norwegians eat fish 3 times a day and have zero heart disease as a result. Although this is a diet that may be one too many herring for most of us, eating it in moderation could be worthwhile. However, you can also get a healthy dose of the omega 3 acids that scrub out your arteries if you lightly oil and briefly grill salmon fillets over high heat. You'll swear the fish is heavily buttered. Serve it with a banana/mango milkshake for a drink to please the kids, but don't tell them they are balancing their menus.

Sample one refinement at a time until you are at ease with it, then mix and match it with your old standbys. Join them in creating new dishes if your teens insist on a vegetarian menu. Most veggie diets are nutritious, balanced, and have been consumed by millions of people for thousands of years, suggesting they aren't quite as boring as meat eaters want us to believe. Don't despair, either, when your little darlings turn up their noses at everything except peanut butter sandwiches. When they can choose from a cafeteria of options, young children eat a balanced diet over time, but not every day. Adults and teenagers who live on diet soda and chips have much less sense. When you've saved gobs of body bucks by trying new, more nutritious foods for the fun of it, consider how to compound your earnings by titillating your taste buds and tickling your nose.

Way back at the base and sides of your tongue lay tiny bumps that lend foods their tastes. Without them, garlic bread tastes like cardboard and spaghetti like wet cardboard. They are marvelous bumps to have although some behave badly and need some tough love before they'll treat you right. Individually, they offer the tastes of salt, sweet, sour, and bitter. The salty ones try their best to be the head honchos, teasing us to shake extra white stuff on our food when most of it already contains all the salt we need. Unless you sweat prodigiously, additional salt swamps our blood streams and contributes to high blood pressure, water retention, and other dis-ease. Uneducated salt buds also mask other tastes that contribute many pleasing flavor combinations to our meals, such as hot and sour, tangy sweet, and sweet sour.

We can train our salt buds to behave more politely by eliminating the extra salt from our menus, a little at a time. If you object that food tastes bland without salt, try low-sodium preparations and seasonings, such as sweet paprika, onion powder, cumin, and garlic powder, or cinnamon and nutmeg. If you like marinara sauce, cook up your own with canned or fresh tomatoes, red wine, a dash of olive oil, garlic, and fennel seed or red pepper flakes. The alcohol in the wine vaporizes, leaving a rich taste and smooth texture with minimal salt. When you waft the rising steam toward you and breathe the wonderful aroma, you'll please your nose, as well as your palate. Garlic powder and a tad of grated Romano cheese perk up low-fat popcorn, sage and poppy seeds pep up noodles, and herbs de Provence (usually a combo of rosemary, thyme, and lavender or basil) brighten almost every dish.

A patient once brought in a shaker of "adobo" seasoning, a complex taste sensation when made from scratch. The label read 95% salt and MSG, 3% drying agent, and a total of 2% of the proper ingredients of adobo: garlic powder, black pepper, anchiote powder, and turmeric. In other words, she bought expensive salt. Read labels. If salt is the first ingredient listed, put the package right back on the shelf. Inspect with care the so-called "healthy" products because some reduced-fat soups contain 20-40% of your total daily salt requirement. Ladling out 2 servings of these is like jumping into a pickling vat. A better choice is to buy dried herbs and spices (cheaper in generic packages) and add them to the fresh foods you prepare from scratch. Sprinkle raw potato slices with onion powder and freshly ground pepper and roast in the oven. Douse asparagus with lemon juice, grate nutmeg on cauliflower, dash onion powder and white pepper on your corn. Your taste buds and your waistline will thank you.

The other pesky taste buds are the sweet ones, as it's difficult to get fat on sour pickles, while bitter taste buds keep nasty things out of our mouths. Sweet buds are natural. Sweet buds are abundant. Sweet buds force brownies and chocolate truffles down our throats. Try fresh fruit instead, for most fruits and vegetables (tomatoes, onions, carrots) contain sugar. Bananas, pears, peaches, and especially grapes are loaded with it. As a bonus, these foods are high in fiber, particularly apples, berries, and oranges. For a quick sugar fix, munch ¼ of a cup of dried fruits: by combining apples, apricots, cranberries, or raisins, you'll end up with a delicious trail mix that will satisfy any sweet tooth. This same mix can be sprinkled on high-fiber cereal for a snack or breakfast. While prunes are the Fort Knox of fiber, eat them dried, not stewed! Be careful not to buy pre-sweetened dried fruits. Let nature's own sweeteners do the job. Canned fruits are convenient and appropriate if you buy the ones packed in low-sugar syrup. Strawberries and raspberries are equally at home on cereal, frozen yogurt, and sponge cake. Have fun thinking up more sugar surrogates that appeal to you while you ring up the body bucks you collect for eating them.

After you've assuaged your salt and sweet buds, take them where they have never gone before. Breakfast on ½ cup of garbanzo beans (chickpeas) sauced with a little olive oil and roasted garlic. Skip the ham and bake your beans with chilies, onions, and cilantro. Sauté bananas or plantains with brown sugar and cinnamon for a superb breakfast or dessert; and dress up fresh fruit salad with a bit of orange juice concentrate and shredded coconut.

Asians chefs understand that a refined diet is both diverse and balanced. They take great care to offer sweet and sour dishes together with spicy and bland ones. To avoid the bite blahs inherent in meals with only one texture, such as chicken ala king over white rice, they are careful to combine crunchy, stir-fried veggies with the smooth textures of chicken or tofu. For extra crunch, slip toasted flaxseed into your muffin batter and scatter the stir-fry with toasted mustard seeds. Hold the mayo and opt for a Thai-style cole slaw made from Napa cabbage sprinkled with vinegar and sugar or sliced cucumbers with rice wine vinegar (or substitute white cider vinegar mixed with sugar and water). Diversify dishes with your eyes by ladling soup into bread bowls or packing fruit salad in hollowed-out orange rind cups. Thrift shops are good places to find cheap, mismatched dishes and silverware for serving pasta on gaudy trays and pita burgers in baskets. Add all the hot sauce or green chilies your tongue can tolerate to pasta or spike yogurt cheese with horseradish for your mashed potatoes. For veggie variety, test the assortment in the organic food sections of your supermarket. Red chard is meaty and white beets don't bleed; parsnips and parsley root turn sweet when steamed. Taste ethnic foods, too: star fruit is pretty on the plate; mangoes and papayas are smooth and sweet; and passion fruit and custard apples are delicately sweet and tart. Eating these foods gives us plenty of nutrients, along with a plethora of tastes and textures.

You probably don't think much about how food smells until your nose meets the vapors arising from a pot of boiling cabbage. Then you learn to revere the aromas emanating from freshly ground coffee beans and bread baking in the oven. Smell is a primitive sense that is essential to most animals though humans pretend it's not important. Because pleasant odors enhance most foods, you might like to sprinkle sage on warm squash or grind cardamom seeds for the carrots. Dill and caraway seeds offer pleasing scents, as do fresh basil, thyme, and rosemary. Grow them on a sunny windowsill or in the summer garden and pop some in your flower arrangements for people to touch and sniff. And you can always rely on the old smell-good trick of baking gingerbread cookies to make your home inviting and cozy. These delicious scents may lighten your mood, as well as make your food taste better.

Considerable research supports the ancient folklore that sniffing lavender soothes the body by relaxing bowel spasms and skeletal muscles. Sniffers solved math problems faster and more accurately, while those who soaked their feet in the herb showed fewer stress symptoms. Lavender also smells good. Regular inhaling of other herbs, better known as aroma therapy, sometimes relieves depression and SAD (seasonal affective disorder). A more dramatic finding is that patients undergoing coronary artery bypass heal faster and experience fewer complications following aroma therapy.

Compulsive Cathy was keen to taste new foods but not salty, lardy, unrefined foods. After her success with homemade veggie chips, she bought an herbal salt substitute for the chips and ate fresh fruit with low-cal yogurt, instead of brownies, for some of her desserts. Once a week, she treated the kids to a Chinese carry out minus MSG, white rice, and deep-fried platters. They were so enchanted by all the remaining choices that they argued about what to order the next time. When they asked her to try new places, she added a vegetarian Indian restaurant, a Japanese sushi bar, a Vietnamese place for do-it-yourself spring rolls, and a Thai spot for curries. No, the kids didn't like the sea urchin eggs but they had fun chasing noodles with chopsticks and slurping their soup Asian style. Being who she was, Cathy tracked her refined diet every day on the computer and jumped on the scales once a week.

She also introduced her children to a secret long used by gourmet chefs: a pretty plate tastes better. The Japanese are masters of delicately sliced vegetables and sushi arranged on a platter as though it's a Picasso canvas. Even their tableware is carefully mismatched to achieve the proper balance. They can make stuffed cabbage rolls look positively elegant. You've probably ordered a dish that looks too good to eat, for 30 seconds, anyway. Practice beautifying your plates with radish and cucumber garnish or stacking the cutlets against a cone of pasta in the center. Pool red pepper sauce under the roast chicken, dash paprika on white things, and look for other ways to give food your personal good looking touch.

On the other hand, Jolly Jim wasn't the least bit interested in chasing computer calories or sampling new cuisines. He was inclined to diminish his diabetes by curbing his confections and cutting back on cocktails with customers. He skipped most restaurant desserts and highballs in favor of club soda with a twist or a wine spritzer poured with equal parts of red wine and club soda that he could nurse through the deal making. When customers insisted on eating chocolate cream pie right in front of him, he ordered fresh fruit to nosh and magically found reasons to wrap up the evening quickly.

Give yourself permission to select foods that match your style, the same way you choose financial investments that suit you. Instead of stuffing your gullet with unimportant junk, refine your menu to maximize your dining pleasure, remembering that the eater's constitution gives you the inalienable right to enjoy your food.

Now that you've thought about food so much that you're having a serious munchie attack, grab a pencil and refine your diet you described in the last chapter. Go into as much detail as you like, or not. This list is a guide, not a demand.

______________________________'s Refined Menu

Your name

My main Wellthy goal is________________________________

To reach this goal, I will (list all that apply)

Join the 200 Club and make $___________body bucks a day

Force out fat by__________________________________

Zap salt by______________________________________

Sample these new foods____________________________

And these new seasonings___________________________

Refine this/these favorite recipes____________________

Refine my family's menu by________________________

Make these food refinements that I've thought of and you haven't ____

CHAPTER 7. IT'S "NATURAL" BUT IS IT GOOD FOR YOU?

For centuries, people have either searched for or peddled the fountain of youth. We've been offered elixirs consisting mainly of alcohol, snake oils allegedly curing everything from hangnails to cancer, and herbs that promise to keep us young and full of life forever. Now, our magic potions are plants alleged to be valuable as medicines or dietary supplements. And everyone from Madison Avenue marketers to movie star entrepreneurs is hounding us to buy natural foods by the fistful.

Your grandmother's chicken soup is natural. The crusty whole grain breads she baked from scratch and the fresh strawberries she scattered on your oatmeal are natural. The ad people don't sell these. They tout products for profit. They attempt to frighten, cajole, and advertise us into buying capsules of garlic, ginkgo, and ginseng. These items and "natural" alfalfa, Echinacea, and valerian come in bottles costing big bucks. A patient once proudly exclaimed that he was taking a natural supplement called "wheat grass" priced at $2.00 an ounce. We were puzzled. Why would he spend so much for dried, processed, and impressively packaged sprouted wheat? He could have sprouted it or alfalfa, lentils, or broccoli at home for pennies. It's easy; just soak the seeds for a day in a jar of water, dump the water, and rinse. Add fresh water to cover the seeds, cap the jar with cheesecloth held by a rubber band, and drain the water. Rinse, water, and drain every day until you see some action. In a few days, your seeds will reward you with plenty of sprouts that are far more nutritious than pills. All kinds of beans are rich in anti-oxidants and sprout easily. Radish and mustard sprouts add a kick to your dishes; black-eyed peas sprouts are packed with calcium; and broccoli sprouts have more vitamin A and C, folic acid, calcium, and iron than their grown up versions.

Natural garlic grows in bulbs under the ground, not in bottles on store shelves. It was used in an amulet to keep evil spirits at bay and still is recommended for zapping cholesterol and mosquitoes. Its unmistakable aroma may render it effective against spirits, insects, and garlic haters when they get a whiff of your breath. Ginger is a lumpy root; ginkgo is a stately tree. Echinacea and valerian grace many gardens with their beautiful flowers and foliage. Feverfew is an attractive chrysanthemum; St. John's wort bears vivid blond flowers, while asclepiads display even more vivid orange ones. These, not the capsules, are the real things.

Ah, but haven't Oriental people and Native Americans used these plants as medicines for centuries? Yes, they have, with one critical difference. Oriental apothecaries dispense fresh and dried herbs, not caplets. Native Americans didn't buy their bergamot in jars; they gathered it from the prairie. Real ginseng and mugwort are a far cry from the bottles offered in stores, as are saw palmetto and skullcap. Ancient and present cultures with a tradition of herbal remedies use plants in their natural state, based on substantial lore and experience. Their value may well stem from the combination of chemicals these plants contain, not from the one substance isolated in pills and diluted with gelatin or oil. If you want to eat naturally, buy the whole food. Don't take cod liver oil in capsules; eat the fish. Feast on a fresh orange or tomato, not a vitamin C tablet; crunch Brazil nuts instead of Vitamin E pills; and peel a banana rather than popping a potassium tablet. A multi-vitamin tablet is handy for the days you nosh on Twinkies when you should dine on turnip greens. However, it is a poor substitute for nature's own vitamin sources. Nature limits how much you can take; man does not. Man tells you 3 pills a day are good for you but 6 are better. Nature tells you an apple a day keeps the doctor away, but don't eat 6 at once; they could make you sick. Nature packages your vitamins complete with cofactors, minerals, and substances yet to be discovered. Nature's own fruits and vegetables come in an assortment of delectable, luscious shapes, colors, and consistencies.

If you do choose to use plants in a pill, do so with caution. Many plants have serious side effects, especially when taken in high doses or in combination with prescription drugs. For example, licorice taken in excess can cause hypertension, low potassium levels, and cardiac arrest. Ginkgo fruit may cause dermatitis, while, for some people, the seeds are toxic. Ginkgo, feverfew, garlic, and ginger can lead to bleeding in people taking coumadin or aspirin. The absinthe in wormwood can kill in heavy doses, as may yohimbe, ma huang, lobelia, and belladonna. To complicate the matter further, some plants (ginseng and guarana) elevate blood pressure, while others (St. John's wort, skullcap) have the opposite effect. Other herbs may augment the effects of prescription drugs with life-threatening consequences. This effect, called confounding, is why most cold remedies containing antihistamines warn you not to combine them with alcohol, lest the nasty results confound you.

Despite this caveat, many plant products are completely benign for most people; and some are truly medicinal. For instance, the heart medication, digoxin, is a synthesized version of the foxglove plant. Hundreds of other plants contain compounds valuable in treating disease. The problem with herbal remedies is that they are like a box of chocolates: you don't know what you are getting until after you've bitten into one. We know little about the interactions of these plants with other substances, the doses that are safe to use, or the types of people who should never take them, such as pregnant women, young children, or people with liver disease. We suggest you study the herbs of interest to you, using neutral references rather than information from the companies selling them. Ask your physician and pharmacist about confounding interactions with prescription drugs you take and make up your own mind. And rest easy. If you have always sprinkled your gumbo with sassafras or laced your pasta sauce with garlic without ill effects, keep up your good eating.

The most natural foods of all can come from your backyard or your windowsill. It may not be a good idea to raise free-range chickens in your apartment, but you can grow terrific tomatoes on your patio. If you have a yard, convert some of the petunias to a pea patch or mingle melons with the nasturtiums and dine on all of them. Brighten your yard with red lettuce or rainbow-colored chard and highlight your daisies with dainty, delicious globe basil. Gardening is fun; and the exercise you get can help in reducing the risk of heart attack, providing the "exercise" is not sitting on a riding tiller. Growing a garden offers a bonus in that you can eat the products of your labor while investing in your health. And where else can you don grubby clothes and silly hats to play in the dirt without scaring off your friends? No yard of your own? Check out community gardens or plots at a local botanic garden if your backyard is a city street. A balcony is a fine spot to plant peppers in pretty pots rimmed with lettuces and radishes, while chives, basil, and thyme flourish on a sunny windowsill. You'll eat the greens and radishes long before the pokey peppers ripen and harvest plenty of herbs to flavor your vinegar and oil salad dressings. Mini tomatoes and purple peppers are cute and colorful in pots on your deck or patio, especially when you pair them with cheery chives and thyme to creep over the edges. Your dividend is that everything in the pots is edible and completely natural when you avoid chemical fertilizers and pesticides.

Since they have dirt in their genes and love to make messes without being scolded, kids are eager to garden. They will delight in "helping" you, particularly when you give each child a few seeds to plant and tend. Big plants suit them. Sunflowers staked and twined with pumpkin vines yield Halloween treats and seeds for the birds. Lash the top ends of stakes together teepee style and plant corn, squash, and pole beans around them to grow a nifty play house. Regale the kids with tales about how Native American Indian farmers grew their crops exactly the same way. Let the kids pick the veggies, too, because nothing is more fun than watching your very own pumpkin grow, until it erupts, spewing seeds and slimy pulp all over the kitchen floor.

Dr. P. scandalized her lawn-loving neighbors by digging up her entire back yard to create an edible herb and vegetable garden. They warmed to the idea when she brought them tender baby lettuces, tomatoes with taste, and cucumbers without wax. Think small. Two or 3 tomato plants yield plenty of fruit for salads and salsa. One squash plant will feed a family of 4 without the produce expanding to the point that the kids make a canoe from it. When your bounty is making you crazy, cook up tomato sauce with your fresh herbs and freeze some in bags laid flat and stacked high. You'll admire your foresight when the snow drifts past your garden window. Frozen herbs bring back the scents of summer at any time of year, so be sure to slip a few into ice cubes for special drinks. When you can't swallow one more veggie, share your wellth. Gather your bountiful beans and cucumbers and take them to the closest food pantry. Those in need will appreciate your gift.

Our grandmas ate natural foods because they tended them in their backyards, or sniffed, shook, and poked them at the market. This is still the custom in cultures where the freshest and finest produce is valued more than cars. You'll appreciate the sentiment when you bite into a ripe tomato picked at its prime. Eat it kitchen sink style, standing over the sink and letting the juices dribble down your chin. But can't we buy fresh tomatoes or apples at the supermarket? No, never. Many store veggies and fruits are gassed, waxed, de-bugged, and held in cold storage for days or weeks. They are rich only in insecticides, fungicides, and chemical fertilizer residue. For instance, tomatoes may be picked green and gassed to appear red in the store. No wonder they are unblemished and tasteless. The organic produce section of your store is a better place to look for natural foods although this term, organic, is puzzling. What is an inorganic plant? The simplest definition is that organic foods are not genetically modified or radiated. They are grown without the use of potentially toxic fertilizers, pesticides, herbicides, and septic sludge. The veggies may not look as good as the gassed stuff simply because they are fresher. They also are more expensive for the same reason. The more consumers demand that standards are enforced for labeling foods as organic, the less we'll be forced to take potluck at the supermarket. Meanwhile, we can patronize farmer's markets and co-ops.

In northern summers, farmers' markets display a dazzling array of delectable produce from artichokes to zucchini, not all of which is organically grown. Some markets allow middlemen to sell Mexican strawberries in Minnesota and Florida peppers in Maine. Ask vendors if these beauties come from up the road or the refrigerator car up the train siding. Your best buys are locally grown, seasonal produce, whether or not it is organically grown. At the least, it is free of banned preservatives and pesticides. And the veggies, not to mention the cheeses and homemade breads at some locations, look so inviting you may come home with enough merchandise to open a café. "You pick" farms and orchards are a good choice for the kids who want to learn about where their food comes from. They will have great fun choosing their own Halloween pumpkin if they didn't raise one themselves.

Another wonderful option is a farm co-op, or community supported agriculture, through which a farmer grows food for a group of shareholders or subscribers, who pay in advance for a portion of the harvest. Ten pounds or so of fresh from the field produce is delivered weekly to common drop points, or you visit the farm to make your selections. Some of these markets plan children's activities and presentations on organic farming or trade produce for your help with the weekly harvest. Others offer free-range chickens, eggs, honey from their own hives, and goat's milk. The cost varies from $600 to $800 per 20-week season for enough veggies to feed a family of 4. You won't get imported sweet corn in April or strawberries in May; but you will collect the best quality and safest food available, plus the satisfaction of preserving the open spaces and styles of small, family farms in your area. Buying from these producers not only assures you of wholesome food, it gives you a say about what you eat. Tell the farmers you want organic, not the cheapest, and most will try to comply with your wishes. If you see kohlrabi and you don't have a clue about how to use it, tell them that, too. To locate farmers' markets, "you pick" farms, and co-ops, contact your county extension service or farm bureau and your community newspapers, or search for local farms on the internet.

I'll try these whole foods to see which of them works for me:

We hope you have so much fun playing with your food that you forget you are chicken walking your way to wellth. Every little step helps, and every effort brings results.

Eating when you are truly hungry, combined with enjoying how your food looks, as well as its aroma, taste, and mouth feel, is an investment that pays terrific dividends, day by day and year after year. One dividend is that, by granting yourself the right to enjoy food for its own sake, you free yourself from the shackles of self-recrimination and guilt that bind you when you try to eat from someone else's plate. Now that you've refined and diversified your eating, you are ready to take the next giant step in building wellth, a step into fit-ease.

CHAPTER 8
FIT-EASE

Each year on January 1, millions of well- intentioned people flock to health clubs, determined to get fit this time, even if it kills them. Their eyes glaze over at the sight of nubile youth with clone-perfect bodies, clad in blinding, neon-colored leotards, jerking, bouncing, and twisting their bodies like living pretzels into positions that would strangle the average person. These fitness-crazed women apparently rely on million-decibel frenetic music to perform their contortions because, when the music stops, they go home. On the opposite end of the room, young men with biceps the size of pickle barrels and legs the width of redwood trees appear to be torturing themselves by trying to lift absurdly heavy circular objects. They grunt and lift, grunt, and clunk down. Every so often, they stop and inspect the pecs of their neighbor to see whose are larger. Other people are doing stranger things with instruments created by descendents of the Spanish inquisition.

Our ancestors labeled such unnatural acts the work of demons and promptly banished these possessed souls to extremely unpleasant fates. Aerobic classes are fine if you have the figure of a high-fashion waif and therefore don't need to attend them. Weight lifting and exercise machines are good if you already have muscles to show off at the gym. They are another matter if you resemble a purple hippopotamus in your new leotard or muscle shirt and move with all the grace of a Sherman tank. Exercise equipment in your home is wonderful, too, if you use it longer than 2 weeks after spending your kids' inheritance to buy it. Within a month, it often transforms into an expensive clothes hanger.

The words "fitness" and "exercise" sound as pleasant to many of us as fingernails raking a chalkboard. They evoke images of running to nowhere like a hamster trapped in an exercise wheel. We prefer the word, "fit-ease" ("fitease" is your new vocabulary word), meaning getting comfortable with moving your body in the style of your choice. Like foodease, fitease comes from defining your present activities and refining them step by step to reach your goals. It goes hand in glove with becoming comfortable with your eating, for it, too, is an investment in your health: your bone, muscular, respiratory, and brain health. It isn't concerned with losing weight, although you may well shed pounds as you become at ease with your body.

Cavemen didn't have to bother with exercise because big hairy creatures intent on eating human sushi for lunch were chasing them. Later, we invented riding lawn mowers and snow blowers to baffle the beasts. We succeeded! The mean critters are gone, along with the best fitness program there ever was, leaving us to grapple with traits inherited from those distant ancestors. Our muscles atrophy when we don't use them; our bodies work overtime storing fat we used to need to survive the next ice age or famine. We suffer mightily when our "fight or flight" adrenaline rush succeeds only in stressing us out because it isn't a good idea to sock a nasty boss or run lickety split away from a scary computer program.

Fortunately, fitease isn't complicated. It's based on the kid's dare, "Bet ya can't rub your stomach and walk backwards at the same time." It requires only that you move your arms and legs simultaneously for as much time as you spend eating dinner. If you inhale your meals, include the time you spend thinking about eating dinner. The idea is to keep going for 30 minutes at a time with no bagel breaks, every day, 5 or 6 times a week. Every ½ hour of activity that increases your heart rate earns body bucks, including mowing the lawn with a push mower, biking 5 miles, raking leaves, walking 2 miles, pushing a stroller 1 ½ miles, swing or other fast dancing, and propelling yourself in a wheelchair, all for ½ hour a day, 5 days a week. Depending on your weight, each of these earns a cool 100-200 body bucks. A 200-pounder collects the top buck, leaving a 125-pound person to take the 100. This is the minimum level of exercise required to maintain your present level of fitness, unless you don't exercise at all, in which case you may earn more than the minimums. Especially if you are out of shape, prolonged exercise is more likely to get you to the ER than to fitease, so don't be tempted to jog 2 ½ hours at a stretch to get it over with.

Most of us exercise by walking to the rest room at work, lugging groceries into the house, or standing in line to buy our fast food breakfast, lunch, and dinner. In some cities, walking on sidewalks is considered downright deviant; the same goes for walking an extra block or up a flight of stairs to a health club.

Working out by scrubbing our floors also is suspect, though hiring a maid to do it so that we may spend more time in our cars and surfing the web is fine. Ironically, our quest to avoid exercise is sickening and killing us by the busload, despite tons of research demonstrating that being fit decreases the incidence of heart disease, ameliorates hypertension, helps control cholesterol, and moderates Type 2 Diabetes. It also reduces the occurrence of colon and breast cancer, stroke, osteoporosis, insomnia, and depression. If these findings fail to impress you, consider that it also improves mental alertness, memory, and mood. The fit among us usually add years to their lives, often years free from the devastation of chronic disease. Yet, in one study, 72% of overweight people who were eager to be fit didn't exercise the recommended minimum of 30 minutes, 5 times a week. Other research confirmed that only 28% of overweight men and women exercised that often. What does it take to lure us away from our computers, SUVs, and remotes for ½ hour a day?

Just as we define and refine our foodease menus, we need a personal fitease menu that suits our histories and goals. When you were a child, was a family outing incomplete without a touch football or volleyball game? Did your parents play tennis or golf? Were you encouraged to play with them, even when you never aced a serve on the court or excelled at finding sand traps on the course? Do you hike and bike with your family or drop them at the skating rink while you catch the football game on the tube? Consider your reasons for wanting to be fit. Do you long to be skinny as a clarinet, flex awesome pecs, don a Brazilian bikini or speedo, or train for a 5k-charity run? Maybe you'd like to stop panting when you climb stairs, be rid of your back pain, or fend off the arthritis that runs in your family.

Your physician may give you a personal set of reasons for being more active, or you may already have a fear that drives you to the gym; a fear that someone stole your toes because you can't see them when you stand up; a panic attack when you discover that your clothes are shrinking in the closet; a fear of flying because the airplane seats are shriveling by the minute. Dr. P. discovered her reason for getting more fit when she noticed that 40-pound sacks of mulch were getting heavier and heavier. She didn't realize that, after age 30, we lose bone and muscle every year, especially after menopause; nor did she expect she would have a problem since she exercised moderately and ate properly, most of the time. When lifting 25 pounds felt like a 100, she signed up for aerobic classes at a community college. The instructors advised her on injury prevention during weight-bearing exercises. The workouts were fun and the camaraderie with her classmates helped keep her in there. Her purpose was to increase muscle mass and bone density so that she could continue with the activities she loved, including hiking, canoeing, and snorkeling. At the very least, she intended to avoid fractures and prevent further deterioration. Later, she added water aerobics because she liked to swim and yoga to improve her balance. Refining her activities in chicken steps brought her closer to her goals. Maintaining fitease is a long term project.

To define your fitease level, add up all the activities you do for 30 minutes a day at a stretch and that seem to increase your heart rate. Dusting the furniture or washing the dishes doesn't count unless you do it at the speed of sound.

I do these activities now for at least ½ hour a day, 5 days a week:

1.____________________________________

2.____________________________________

3.____________________________________

If you exercise less than ½ hour a day, why?

Check all that apply.

___I don't have time.

___I'm too tired.

___I'm too old.

___I'm too fat.

___I'm too out of shape.

___Exercise hurts.

___I have a bad back.

___Exercise is boring.

___I'll make a fool of myself.

___I can't afford the expense.

___My grandmother never exercised and she lived to be 100.

___My other excuses are___________________________________.

Our reasons for not becoming minimally fit are highly creative although not always accurate. Let's take the "no time" excuse that most people fall back on because we ARE extremely busy with our careers, families, and endless chores. Make fitness, not folding the laundry, a priority and do 2 things simultaneously every chance you get. Check out Timewraps for ideas on the subject.

Too tired, old, fat, or flabby? Experts shout loudly and clearly that exercise improves our health, no matter what shape we're in when we start. Consult an advisor about activities you can do safely if you have a bad back, knee, or any other infirmity. When you get bored, try another activity (sky diving, anyone?). You're bound to find something you enjoy doing. You say that you can't afford to exercise? Jog around your neighborhood, speed walk at the mall, and lift weights in your bedroom. If you're self-conscious about your appearance or afraid you can't keep up with the group, choose activities for which you can keep your clothes on and workout among people with similar abilities. Loners and competitive people may be most comfortable exercising at home. Like the Dow-Jones, fitness data are averages and may not apply to every specific individual, as we enter the health club from diverse environments and gene pools. It's important to think about your future years. Will you be happy rocking on the porch and watching TV when you retire?

One way to ease your way to fitness is to create a personal fitease spa at home. A home health club is convenient, familiar, and comfortable. It may ruin your favorite excuse of having no time to exercise. Install any or all of these toys: TV, radio, CD/DVD player, telephone, bookstand, or headphones. Tape the soaps for viewing during your exercise time, swap ball game scores with your friends; sing along with your favorite tunes. Use your retreat for stretching, step aerobics, yoga, or belly dancing. When you get winded, quit the crunches and dance.

If you feel winded, slow down a bit to take your pulse to insure that your heart is keeping pace with your arms and legs. Feel your pulse on your wrist or neck for 20 seconds and multiply this number by 3 to get your heart rate per minute. You can find information on your maximum heart rate at http://www.americanheart.org/presenter.jhtml?identifier=4736. You are looking for a heart rate at least 50% of maximum or a rate of 85-144 beats per minute in the above example. A rate higher than that will get you to the ER; a lower rate means your heart's not in it. Remember, fitease is a long term project. Gradually build your endurance and you will accomplish your goals.

Wanting to lose his extra pounds, Jolly Jim hopped off his golf cart and started carrying his own bags on his weekly foursome with customers. When he was on the road, he patronized hotels featuring exercise rooms and made it a habit to work out for ½ hour every morning. This combination bought him a whopping 2400 body bucks a week. But, after awhile, he complained, "Since losing the first 15 pounds, I've lost only 3 pounds in the past 2 weeks. What am I doing wrong?" Jim should have been overjoyed, as it's healthiest to lose 1 or 1 ½ pounds a week. Much of an initial drop in weight is water, but keep drinking plenty of it anyway because racing to the bathroom every ½ hour is good exercise. A rapid weight loss may not be beneficial since it might include stuff you want to hang on to, such as muscle.

When Compulsive Cathy investigated her fitness options, she discovered in-line skating. She earned far in excess of her 200 body bucks a day while she and the kids had fun tearing around the neighborhood. Cathy met several new people, including a single dad who invited her over for burgers with their combined families.

"That's fine for her," you may mutter. "Geraniums can skate better than I. If I fall, it will take all day to pick up the pieces." Cathy chose an activity she enjoyed- - slowly. At first, she skated a leisurely 10 minutes, gradually working up to an hour at a time after dropping the kids off with a neighbor when they tired. If you can't skate but you can play ping pong, practice as fast and as often as you can. Or head over to an alley to bowl 10 lines. If you love the outdoors, dust off your golf clubs and play 9 holes to start. Gardening is fun. Grab a hoe and weed all the gardens on the block. If sports aren't your style, go dancing; the faster the better. Square dancing is quick, polkas are quicker; and waltzing adds elegance to your exercise. The Viennese try to keep it a secret, hoping no one discovers that waltzing the night away in dress-up clothes is an elegant high.

After you've decided what you expect to gain from an exercise program, outline a program in your style, constantly refining your activities to meet your goals. Try to include a few new activities you'd like to try, as well as the exercise you get now for at least the minimum ½ hour a day. Give yourself permission to enjoy your body by picking and choosing activities you like. Your purpose is to invest in your body in ways that build wellth while indulging in pastimes you enjoy.

______________________________'s REFINED FIT-EASE MENU

My 2 primary fitness goals are: (One should be to earn at least 200 body bucks a day if you're not already at this level.)

1.____

2.____

I will refine my current menu with these activities:

____

____

____

____

In 6 months, I'll review my status and goals, revising them as necessary.

Congratulations! Now you can collect more body bucks by compounding the interest on your fitease investments.

CHAPTER 9.
FITEASE DIVIDENDS

Bonnie Biker hadn't paid much attention to exercising. What bothered her was her eating. She had been 35 pounds overweight for as long as she could remember, despite going on a new diet at least twice a year and always dropping 10 pounds or so until the goodie goblins attacked. With a couple of weeks of giving in to coffeecake and caramels, she weighed as much as when she started. She didn't find it amusing to see a pumpkin in the mirror nor did she enjoy having to lie down to zip up her jeans. It's no fun either to go shopping in disguise lest our friends spot us in the king or queen-size departments. With consistent exercise, we'll look better even if we don't lose weight; and isn't that the point? Fat wouldn't be so hard to handle if no one could see it. By increasing our muscle mass and decreasing the flab, nobody will guess that we inhaled a couple of jelly donuts when no one was looking. Picture an empty air mattress, a lumpy blob until it's inflated. Muscles firm and tidy our appearance like the air in that mattress.

The next time Bonnie got the diet urge, she jumped on her bicycle instead. Along with refining her breakfast menu by eating 1 less slice of cheesecake, she pedaled to the park for an hour 3 days a week, alternating with an hour of brisk walking on the other 3 days. A year later, she was 25 pounds lighter and so firm that the extra 10 pounds vanished under her new muscles. Bonnie learned to balance her craving for goodies with activities she liked, choosing to pedal away some of the double fudge brownies she loved rather that giving all of them up. Being in charge of her fitease goals, she said, was both empowering and satisfying. Bonnie earned her fitease dividend by saving body bucks from exercising, rather than by severe dieting.

You may have envied a youthful-looking, svelte acquaintance until you discovered, much to your chagrin, that he/she was older and heavier than you. Before you ask people like this what kind of corsets they wear, look at amateur athletes. They are nearly always heavier than they appear because they have a much higher ratio of muscle to fat than do couch potatoes. Since we associate slim physiques with youth, they also appear younger without the bother of tummy tucks and facelifts. The ones in shoulder pads and facemasks don't count. All of them look like King Kong anyway.

Does this mean it's not necessary to cut back on calories and fat if I exercise enough? You're right. You don't, depending on your definition of "enough." Triathletes burn so many calories they can scarf down an entire peach pie ala-mode every day if they like. But they don't. To maximize their performance, athletes are fussier than most about balancing their menus and seldom overdose on fat and sugar. They also train 2-6 hours a day, 6 or 7 days a week, a version of "enough" that would drive most of us non-mountain men right to the cookie jar. A better refinement is to earn 200 bucks a day by eating slightly less and 200-300 more by increasing the intensity or duration of your workouts.

Biking wasn't Ellie Extrovert's style. At age 45, she weighed 195 pounds that, at 5" tall, was not acceptable. She tried a gamut of diet plans and they all worked, for a while. Ellie joined a health club; but, for a variety of reasons, she seldom worked out there. What she liked was fast dancing at noisy clubs among crowds of people. After 3 weeks of rocking, she lost 2 pounds. Within 6 months, she got rid of the pain from an inflammation of her chest-wall lining. Her husband slimmed down, too, for a grand total of 100 fewer pounds in 3 years. The only bad part was that Ellie couldn't crack any more jokes about their having 10 tons of fun in bed. This was a small price to pay for Ellie and her husband's fitease.

Maybe hitting a tennis ball is a problem because, when you do, loud creaking noises emanate from your knees, back, and neck. Often this "rusty hinge" effect results from muscles weakened by inactivity and age-muscles in need of gentle stretching to increase their flexibility. If your knees screech when you try to squat, do a slow, half squat 10 times a day to reacquaint them with their duties. Simple stretching exercises, as in reaching for the sky, beginning yoga routines, and T'ai chi, are useful for limbering up and improving balance. T'ai chi is practiced by a billion or so people around the world. It helps unfit people to breathe deeply and improve their balance. One study found that elderly people reduced their falls by 47% after they practiced regularly. Most said they felt calmer and more serene following T'ai chi sessions as though their spirits, as well as their bodies, were better balanced. Another option for the soon-to-be fit is "aquacise," which is calisthenics and aerobic routines performed in the swimming pool. It offers most of the benefits of dry exercise while sparing the joints.

Exercises, such as these, are strongly encouraged by members of the American College of Sports Medicine folks, who previously demanded all manner of cruel and unusual punishment in the name of fitness. Now the sports people say that the catchy phrase, "Go for the burn" refers to rockets. And "No pain, no gain" should be left to aspiring martyrs like those in the 14th century who wore clothes of thorns which they beat on to prove their faith or maybe to keep warm. These sports people advise us that it's important to just go with the slow flow. They also point out that every tiny chicken step you take counts. If you can't manage aerobics, do what you can and continue doing it. You will get comfortable with your body though it will take you longer to reach the level of fitness that you desire. Your body is wonderfully adaptable. It will learn any activity you teach it, given time. Ease into shape slowly.

This point is especially encouraging for mid-life women who may be unfit and overweight. Ladies, this is not always the case. You may still have a wonderful shape but still be out of shape. Or you may still have a great shape and be in great shape. In that case, continue doing all of the great healthy and "Wellthy" things you already are while incorporating some new ones. However, while no one knows why, it is certain that expecting to be out of shape contributes to becoming out of shape. Substantial research suggests that both men and women can and do achieve fitease at any age. When you expect to be active at age 60 or 80, you amble in the park, jump in the lake, snorkel with the grandkids, bogie on the greens. You also compound the benefits with a special dividend of enhanced brainpower. Not only does regular aerobic activity stretch your life span, it enhances performance on tests of reasoning and recent memory, two areas in which older people often feel they are deficient. This makes sense as memory loss and lack of exercise are associated with heart disease and diabetes, in addition to poor health in general. You can take pleasure in knowing that you are piling up brain bucks while you pile on the muscles when you exercise.

Here's another dividend of fitease. Try as hard as you can to get prodigiously upset while you are furiously pedaling your bike or attempt to weep buckets of tears while swimming full speed ahead. It won't work. It's impossible to stay stressed out during vigorous activity, no matter how hard you want to have a bad day. If you are extremely annoyed with the boss, beat on a punching bag. A quick turn around the block may keep you from shouting at the kids, while shooting baskets could completely wipe out memories about the last argument you lost with your spouse. And you will feel better for it.

Within a year of starting daily aerobic activity, you may, while exercising at your peak, feel like laughing out loud. In fact, you may go ahead and guffaw. An appointment with your shrink is not indicated. Runner's high is tickling your brain with happy chemicals called beta-endorphins. These lovely substances result in incredibly pleasant experiences ranging from contentment to an intoxicating kind of elation. Or, you may experience similar changes if you are severely oxygen-deprived. Dr. P. met runner's high (or lack of CO2) while swimming long distance. After miles of ocean and after catching her "second wind"- yes, this, too, is a real experience stemming from the release of epinephrine- she imagined she was a small planet drifting weightlessly through space. It was a charming thought for a chubby teenager. This was far more inspiring than thinking about sea monsters nibbling her toes which was what she had been thinking about to push past exhaustion.

Most athletes pretend they have no idea what you're talking about when you mention athletic euphoria to them. Apparently, they want to keep a good thing to themselves because they say things like "Exercise makes you feel better." It certainly does. Why do you suppose more long-distance runners report that they think about running while having sex than think about sex while running? When pressed, many compulsive exercisers admit they work out specifically to get high- cheaply and legally. And you might, too.

In case you haven't noticed, another way to feel good is to have sex. Not only is it good for you emotionally, it puts bucks in your 200 Club. In research on 2500 men, 45 to 59 years of age, the more sexually active subjects (intercourse twice a week or more) died at half the rate of the sexually inactive ones the same age. The survivors may have been healthier to begin with, though other studies with both sexes reveal that having sex raises good cholesterol, reduces aches and pains including those pesky headaches, tunes up the prostate, and increases production of feel-good hormones. We trust you can find other reasons for having sex, but it may please you to know that 15 minutes of active intercourse earns 50 to 100 body bucks that, at twice a week, sheds 1 ½ to 3 pounds a year. What a bonus!

Walking is a fine way to get fit, partly because most of us can do it regardless of how old, fat, and decrepit we are. It is, by no means, the best exercise for you; but, if it is all you can do, do it. After a while, you'll be able to do more. Do what feels good. Climb up cliffs, paint the house, or punch a volleyball. If you like to feel you've accomplished something, try activities that get you somewhere, such as canoeing, hiking, or weeding your garden. It's difficult to boast that you rowed 5 miles in your living room or climbed a thousand steps in your one-level home when you'd rather be rowing on the river and rock climbing in the Adirondacks. On the other hand, pumping bicycle pedals isn't a good idea if you don't know how to ride. Try dog paddling in the pool instead. Pick activities you can do close to home as it makes more sense to swim than ski if the nearest snow is 5 days away. Curling and ice-skating don't work well in Alabama; and, unless you love to sing in the rain, jogging in the park isn't much fun in Seattle winters. Great results can come from modest beginnings.

Doris Desperate was a new mom, age 31, who hated exercise and weighed in at 50 too many pounds. She enrolled in an expensive weight-loss program, ate no more than the meals she was given, not cheating even once. They refunded her money. Doris failed to lose a single pound after several months of starvation dieting on a regime "guaranteed" to take it off. Even as a child she had never been active. She felt like a klutz just thinking about sports. Her style was wandering around malls, poking her head into shops to try on clothes and dream about how she would look in an outfit 3 sizes smaller. Completely frustrated, she strapped on a baby carrier and walked with her daughter for a slow ½ hour to start. Trekking with a 20-pound load was tiring at first; but, within a month, she stretched her time to 45 minutes and doubled her speed with no window shopping until she was done. She lost 4 pounds in the first month.

Tony Tubby was a 14 year old, massively overweight couch potato. He was the brunt of every bad joke in school. Exercise was impossible, or so he thought. His doctor taught him "T.V." exercises which were to be done at home. The only rule was that he had to spend 1 hour watching T.V. daily. Tony agreed though he knew nothing would work. During the first commercial, Tony did as many crunches as he could (6 the first day). The second commercial required push-ups, the third, leg raises. The cycle then started over again until the hour ended. At the end of 3 months, Tony was seeing results. He reveled in competing with himself. By the end of the first year, no one laughed at Tony. The now strapping 15 year old was playing high school football.

To combat the ho-hums, try diversifying your activities, alternating window washing with walking your dog or badminton with biking. Athletes call this "cross training," valuable for strengthening different muscles and for preventing both brain and muscle boredom. Muscles adapt readily to almost every activity and tell us so by putting the brakes on our metabolism. Trick them into speeding up again by changing their jobs on a day to day basis. Go from playing bocce ball to bowling, or handball to horseback riding. Stringing different activities together at faster and faster paces also gives you the benefits of aerobics without actually feeling like you are exercising. If you can vacuum the house and the cat at 50 miles an hour with time to spare, all the better for you (not so good for the cat).

For a time, you lift weights and sweat, jog with the dog and sweat, play killer racquetball and sweat, and refine your food menu to match. It works. In 3 months, you've lost 12 pounds, your abs are flatter, your deltoids stronger. You are so full of yourself you expect to resemble a world-class body builder/ super model in 3 more months. A week passes, then another. The bathroom scales must be broken because they read the same. Your waistline measures the same, even when you suck it all in. The doctors must be lying. You want to dive into the banana cream pie and die there. This dastardly event is called a plateau. It feels like you've hit a stone wall. It slams most people despite the fact that they are shedding pounds and/or adding muscle. It happens because our bodies are programmed to preserve as much of ourselves as possible, lest we get stuck in another ice age. We adjust to less food and more exercise by slowing our metabolism to conserve the energy we may need to fight off mastodons. When you notice biking 20 miles was impossible 3 months ago but now you aren't even winded, you've banged smack into a plateau. It occurs even when we are losing weight and exercising in safe, gradually increasing increments, and it is not fair. The best solution is to stay off the scales and put away tape measure for a couple of weeks while you up your exercise ante. Increase a 30- minute, 2-mile walking pace to 2 miles in 24 minutes, or stride for 45, and then 60 minutes without stopping for latte.

On alternate days, lift weights, shoot baskets with the kids, or treat them to a canoe ride. This cross training will eventually kick-start your performance to a higher level, but be patient. For many of us, the last 5 or 10 pounds don't want to leave our side, literally. Here are some ways to climb down from your mesa (don't expect instant results). As with any exercise, if you feel nauseated, dizzy, weak, or in pain, or hear the grass talking, exercise your good judgment and STOP!

Now is the time to think about your Body Bucks. It doesn't matter whether you use your Play Money (remember, Play $$$ = No Handcuffs from Treasury Agents) or your check register of deposits per day.

ACTIVITY	Calories earned per hour per weight	
	200 lbs.	130 lbs.
Baseball	380	230
Canoeing	560	350
Foursome golf	330	200
Rock climbing	850	500
Soccer	730	450
Tennis, fast	800	490
Walking 2 mph	280	175

Just as you have a financial advisor to guide your monetary investments, your physician can help you grow both your foodease and fitease investments. The keystone for both is an annual physical exam that includes procedures he/she may recommend, such as mammograms for women and prostate exams for men over age 50.

As you age, you may want to reduce your caloric intake and switch to lower impact activities. Unless you are a lumberjack, you probably don't require the infinite calories from gallons of milk, pepperoni pizzas, and all the other junk inhaled by teenagers. Going out for the football team isn't such a good idea either. Men seem to be more reluctant than women to visit a physician when they aren't sick; so wise up, guys. Hypertension, diabetes, prostate cancer, kidney and liver disease, to name a few, can be detected only by a medical exam. A regular check-up helps to preserve your physical assets. Just as a wise investor reviews his financial portfolio on a regular basis, you need to review your physical/nutritional assets yearly. Let your physician be your fitease investment counselor. After you've met your first-year goals, prepare a wish list of the activities you want to be doing in 5, 10, and 20 years from now and/or what you plan to do after you retire. Do you want to go scuba diving within a year? Play tennis at age 75? Or will you be playing only bingo by then? Because your immediate goals may dictate what you will be enjoying 30 or 40 years from now, you may want to test drive several options over the next year or 5 or 10. Here's a sample list:

In one year, I will learn to ride a horse.
In 5 years, I will take a horseback riding tour of Germany.
When I'm 55, I'll hike part of the Pyrennes from France to Portugal.
At age 65, I'll swim and snorkel the Bay Islands of Honduras.
At age 75, I'll go on a walking tour of Wales.

At age 80, I'll take a whale-watching cruise off Baja.

Feel free to quit listing at the age you wish you could live to and still be in good health.

_____________________________'s WISH LIST

In a year, I will____

Five years from now, I will______________________________

Ten years from now, I will_______________________________

At age 65, I will_______________________________________

At age 75, I will _______________________________________

At age 85, I will ____

CHAPTER 10.
SELF-EASE

Take a look at your thumb. Either thumb will do as long as it's attached to your hand. Pick up this book using that thumb and your fingers. Notice how your thumb and fingers cooperate to lift the book. Can you lift it with just your thumb? Can you do it using only your other fingers? Maybe so, but it's terribly awkward and why are we doing this?

Children love to draw faces on their fingertips and pretend they are people. Try drawing on your fingers or trace your hand on paper and draw on it if you have a fear of colorful fingertips. It's OK to act like a kid. Put your face on your thumb as best you can, then draw your spouse or other special person on your index finger. Put a significant friend on your middle finger and a colleague from work on the fourth digit. On your little finger, draw the face of someone from a group to which you belong, maybe your church, parent association, professional society, or lodge. If none of these apply, draw the cashier at a supermarket. Depict your children's faces on your other hand or on your toes if you begot more than four. Save the thumb on that hand for your secret self, that part of your self-ness you shelter from everyone because it's too personal to reveal. If your children are watching you as though you've gone bananas, invite them to draw their own set of faces, and let their fingers do the talking.

Just as we need our fingers and thumb to grasp a book comfortably, we rely on positive relationships with our lovers, families, friends, and coworkers. Our self-ness, like a thumb that works in opposition to the other fingers, represents our individuality as unique as a thumbprint. To have good relationships with others, we first need to feel comfortable in our own heads. Let's call this kind of comfort "self-ease." Feeling at home with yourself isn't as simple to measure as your weight or temperature, though it's just as real in its consequences for your health. Constantly feeling angry, hating your body, or feeling inadequate can lead to overeating, high blood pressure, and belly aches. Our immune systems crumble when negative emotions persist too long and we get sick. Not only is self-ease ("selfease" is the new vocabulary word") a lot more fun than feeling stressed or scared or useless, wellth depends every bit as much on selfease as it does on our financial, food, and fitness investments. Test your selfease by moving to a quiet place with no TV, phone, radio, or kids. Do nothing for half an hour. What did it feel like? Some people delight in their own company; others avoid it like peanut butter and anchovy sandwiches. Some of us think we can't take time out at all. The kids have to get their shots; the canary has a cavity. Maybe so, but investing in yourself pays dividends at least as great as your financial investments. You won't take pleasure in your financial wealth if depression or envy cripples you.

It's a pleasure to have 54-year old Do Dat Dan as a patient. When he developed cancer of the tongue that required surgery and radiation therapy, he endured both without complaining. Despite losing his sense of taste and finding it difficult to swallow, his response to each hardship was, "We can do dat." When the radiation completely exhausted him, he said, "We can do dat" and went back to work wearing turtlenecks to cover the angry scar down the side of his neck. His positive attitude never changed, even when people stared at his gaunt appearance and the bright red rash on his face. It didn't change when his live-in girlfriend left him for a younger, healthier person. After 5 years in remission, Dan is still proudly doing "dat." We hope he lives to be 100 because he takes charge of his health instead of hiding behind his pain and fatigue. Yes, it's hard to find the time to prepare whole food meals and get fit, much less to take 10 for ourselves. But we can do that, too, using our 200 Club cash. Take 200 seconds (3 ½ minutes) a day to do your thing, whether it is combing the iguana or meditating, or meditating while combing the iguana. Both reduce stress although the iguana may be confused. Add 200 Body Bucks to your Club total each day you de-stress your way. These bucks aren't calories saved but are equally important minutes added to your life.

To be contented with being you, you need to be selfish by nurturing your self-ness. Begin by applying the golden rule to yourself. Do unto you as you would have others do unto you. Take time off from incessant family, work, school, and community demands to spend your Club 200 time your way. Define how you want to spend your alone time and refine it as required. Use your private time to work on a puzzle, pitch a Frisbee, or plant a petunia. Take a bubble bath, dye your hair orange, or read through dinner. Or do nothing at all.

Feel free to spend your selfease time in your style, the same as you choose to eat and exercise. Our sole suggestion is that you pick solitary activities that relax and comfort you like a crackling fire on a bitter winter night. No fair carving peach pits to sell or practicing pool shots to whip the neighbor who always whips you. Whittle or weave because it pleases you, not to collect another buck or gold star. Stress and flex in your private exercise space. Brew a cup of herbal tea and meditate. Dig into a trashy paperback, stitch needlepoint, or hurl darts. Take off your shoes and snooze. Turn up the Beethoven, the guided imagery tape or R&B, if the latter is more your style, and commit oemphalopsychism (contemplation of one's navel). Both music and meditation reduce anxiety, lower blood pressure, and slow heart rate; and you won't even sweat. Don't know how to meditate? Inhale from your abdomen and say "ten" as you exhale deeply enough to make your belly stick out. Repeat 10 times or until you are dizzy or need a bathroom. Do you think that because you are an important person you've no time for this nonsense? Because you are an important person, you need to make time for this "nonsense."

A majority of retired executives from IBM, 3M, and the like said they would spend more time in contemplation if they could repeat their lives. They also said they would take more risks, especially in love and work, the second time around. Finishing this book or the birdhouse you're building isn't important. Sensing how you breathe, how the room smells, and feeling your body are the important things. Don't retire with regrets; reflect instead on the big picture, the panorama of your life, and skip the mini crises of the day. You aren't wasting time or neglecting your responsibilities. You are building a self better equipped to deal with external pressures, such as eating one potato chip. Feel free go to the movies one afternoon, walk the dog for an hour the next, and practice your piccolo on the third. Doing what pleases you, not what your lover or kids or boss want you to do, lends a whole new meaning to the phrase, "I'm enjoying my 'self'."

Another way to enjoy your "self" is to pursue an interest or hobby, one that may or may not involve other people. If you are passionate about bagpipes, by all means practice on them and march in more parades. If you don't care for kilts, challenge yourself by learning a new skill that intrigues you. Diversify your self-investments and take zither lessons if you don't know how to strum, learn to yodel if you can't sing a note, or practice public speaking if you want to perfect your timing in telling jokes. If you would rather eat maggots than step on a podium, consider taking a course in Sanskrit, joining a book discussion group, or starting a coin collection. University researchers urge us to exercise our brains by first turning the TV off. Dust off the scrabble board, work a crossword puzzle, or challenge a worthy opponent to a game of chess. Reading anything, even the comics, pumps up your brain and keeps it forever youthful. These findings resulted from a long-term study of nearly 6000 older people, 70% of whom stayed mentally sharp, particularly those who had a passion. Poor health, not aging, was to blame for the foggy memory and sloppy reasoning we often associate with old age. Clearly, investing in our brain, as well as the rest of our body, pays significant dividends.

Visualize acquaintances that love to sit for hours painting, ride Harleys, or run marathons on the treadmill in the basement. Do they seem happy with them "selves?" Yes! People with interests beyond work and family are usually rich in optimism and self-ease. You won't feel depressed while you're leaping to net a swallowtail butterfly or when you've taught your cat to bark. Pride and self-confidence are guaranteed every time you nurture a knockout gorgeous orchid, build a computer with the kids (one that actually works), or find that silver-plated bed pan you've always wanted. Interests are warm fuzzies for your spirit. They make you feel good for the doing of them, even when your clarinet screeches or your prize cockroach croaks. They sustain wellth for a lifetime, a point illuminated by findings that healthy, retired executives don't retreat into the TV. Instead they continue to pursue their passions, some by consulting part-time with their former employers, others by mentoring people who covet their knowledge of business.

We suspect that people who lack self-esteem are people who lack a passion. These people probably aren't very interesting because they aren't interested, as opposed to those who can earn their livings doing what they love. To feel good about your self, get an interest, get involved, and get going.

Moneybags Mike was the antithesis of an involved person. At 40, he owned a mortgage-free mansion, 3 cars, and a yacht. Making more money was his passion, his purpose in life. In his spare time, he counted it and told himself how superior he was. He didn't care to read or travel. He didn't surf the net or do anything he could pay someone else to do. He drank too much and caught colds frequently.

Mike said he would feel better when he bought his second home. Initially money was a vehicle Mike used to take him somewhere. Money became his destination. Mike saved all his money and spent all of his wellth and his health. His immune system failed when he developed pneumonia and he died at the age of 55.

Do you want to perk up your immune system, zap some fat, and slam the brakes on aging? You can do all 3 free of charge with no sweat any time you like and have a ball doing it. It may sound like a fountain of youth but it isn't. It's a laugh. Literally. A holding-your-sides belly laugh with tears streaming down your cheeks is best but even a modest chuckle reduces stress. Study after study reveals the healing power of laughter. The immune function of college students soars after they view funny videos, seriously ill patients improve more rapidly when they are treated to live slapstick in the hospital, and patients who laughed more before they became ill survived cancer at a higher rate than those who didn't. These findings are so pervasive that hospitals conduct laugh-therapy groups for outpatients, as well as silly seminars where their employees can put on clown suits and cut up. Catching your breath after you hoot at a good joke and then breathing deeply because you are pumping as much oxygen to your brain as a brisk walk is a great stress reliever, as well. In addition, both laughter and walking stimulate memory and problem solving skills, especially in older folks.

Because laughing, like other exercise, releases happy endorphins that elevate your mood long after you stop, don't fret when you want to keep on guffawing. Each chortle and chuckle contributes to your very happy Club 200. If you've forgotten how to laugh hard and many of us have, practice smiling. Search every day for a funny or sweet happening that makes you grin or giggle. It may be as cozy as a cat snuggling her kittens or as exuberant as a small boy resolutely steering a parked car. It can be hearing a terrific new joke or reading the kids a Dr. Seuss story. It might be as simple as catching yourself doing something stupid and having the self-confidence to laugh at it. From porky pig to puns, anything that tickles you is a winner. Take advantage of your private time to view a comedy video or TV program that amuses you. Listen to tapes of old radio programs or read a funny novel. Trade silly jokes with the children and join their nonsense games. Because kids laugh at everything and invent fun every chance they get, the sound of their jubilance might infect you if you let it. Hone your humor at a comedy club or chat with a humor group on the Internet. The more you smile and laugh, the happier you'll feel because acting happy tends to trigger a flood of positive emotions. Finding a funny event the day your house burns down can be a problem, and you might not care to laugh out loud at a funeral. Otherwise, you will uncover mirth all around you, and in you, if you look. You'll know when you are collecting selfease dividends because you'll like your "self" better. Other people will sense it, too, as you become more pleasant to be around.

CHAPTER 11.
PEOPL-EASE

Will Rogers was wrong when he said, "I never met a man I didn't like." Some people are as pleasant as sticking needles under your fingernails. They are tongue-lashing tyrants who should be tossed in a tar pit and needle-some gnats to be squashed forthwith. No doubt you have your own list of babbling bores and whining wimps who peeve and pester you.

Picture yourself inside a giant soap bubble in a cluster of bubbles that overlap. Each bubble represents one of the social roles you play and encompasses all the people with whom you interact in that role, whether it is mom, friend, spouse, or colleague. No matter how hard we try, there's no way we can perform all our roles, all the time, to the satisfaction of other people. Sometimes we can't perform them to our own satisfaction and our bubble bursts.

Most nights, Menopausal Mona thrashed fitfully and had to pry herself out of bed in the morning. Her hot flashes weren't too bad, but she burst into tears or snapped at her husband for no reason anyone could imagine. He told her he couldn't take having a "sweet as apple pie" wife one day and a shrew the next and moved into the guestroom. She didn't have to cook for a crowd anymore because her college aged kids came home only to get 6 months of laundry done. Her husband, at the height of his career, stayed late at his penthouse office most nights and golfed with his associates on weekends. Waiting for him at night, Mona plopped in front of the TV and stuffed her face, hating herself for putting on the weight. What could be wrong? She wondered.

Estrogen supplements vanquished most of Mona's hot flashes, while a mild anti-depressant ameliorated her insomnia. These symptoms were easy to mend but they weren't the main problem. As a homemaker who hadn't been employed since her marriage, Mona's bubbles as mother, wife, and tireless school volunteer had burst. She needed new roles to replace those that had occupied her for 25 years. While mulling over what to do next, she volunteered in the cardiac rehab unit of her local hospital where a nurse suggested she'd make a good rehab technician. Intrigued, Mona enrolled in the program offered by a nearby community college. She liked her courses enough to take more the next semester, and the next. Following an internship at the college rehab facility, she graduated with an AA degree. Within a year, she was thrilled to accept an invitation to head the rehab lab where she had interned. Mona likes her job because she feels she is making a difference in her new roles as employee, boss, and co-worker. Though still whittling her weight down, she is rid of her insomnia and hot flashes. She's earning big body bucks by leading her patients' exercise sessions 5 days a week. She schedules a special date with her husband every week for the two of them to rediscover how to have fun together as they did before the children arrived. He, in turn, is back in the marital bed and tries hard to tell her every day that he loves her.

We cannot possibly be equally competent parents, children to and sometimes caretakers of our own parents, best friend to our lovers or spouses, and good friend of others while spending 10 hours a day building our careers. The key to this dilemma is to decide what you want to do the most and send it to the top of your list. If you throw up at the thought of changing diapers, don't stay home with the babies. Your children are better off with a nanny or loving day care environment if you are so bored by baby talk that you watch talk shows all day. When you miss spending time with your lover, leave your briefcase at the office and step out with your special person. Talk to your mom when you aren't obligated to call her. Say no to your neighbor who asks you to black top her driveway, to the kids when they beg for rides to lion-taming practice because they don't feel like walking 10 minutes to get there, to your mother-in-law when she pressures you to take her alligator hunting because she doesn't drive. Begin each day by asking your "self:" "Who are the most important people in my life? Who will be there in 10 years? Who would I miss most if he or she were gone?" Choose to invest most of yourself in the people who make this list and continue to refine your "self" time that is invested in people pleasing. We don't want to lose our real "self" time because we are trying to please and accommodate everyone else.

Dr. P. once asked her elderly father how he managed to sustain a happy marriage for over 50 years. He said there were 3 important ways: compromise, compromise, and compromise.

Take his advice if you can, especially if troublesome people occupy your house. Happy people bring out the best in you. They make you feel smarter, funnier, and nicer. You want to bring out their best, too; and you shall. Tell them your funny story of the day, especially when the joke's on you. We much prefer to hear how other people make fools of themselves than when we do. You'll seem supremely human and you may collect a bunch more funny stories to chuckle about.

Families that laugh together stay together, particularly when the adults know how to play. No, we don't mean tennis. Watch your young children; they know how to play. They have fun for hours with cardboard boxes, pots and pans, rhymes and riddles. Mud puddles and dirt are even better. When you use your imagination and refuse to take yourself seriously, you, too, can play. Set aside 200 seconds a day to put on ridiculous hats, play your music from way back, and dance with your kids, your partner, or the broom. Teach your children silly songs and trade knock-knock jokes. They will find you irresistible.

When it rains, take them to websites you've surfed and approved. These might be interactive games, coloring pages, their school sports events, or fodder for a term paper on the Samoan constitution. At the dinner table, talk about their day; plan a family bike outing, a trip to a planetarium, or a laser show. Any event new to all of you will do, such as swimming in molasses. Join in their computer games until they win every time, then switch to something you can win like watermelon seed-spitting contests. When they fall in love with dinosaurs, take turns drawing murals depicting fierce, ugly ones. Let the kids cook dinner; and, when necessary, pretend you love it. Investigate the native Americans who lived at your place as an entrée to roasting corn, growing pole beans, or smoking pemmican the way they once did, perhaps in your own backyard. Schedule family activities. When your teenagers would rather dash to the ball field than spend one more minute with a parent, take comfort that they're getting fit and tucking away memories that will live on in stories to their children. Whether they demand it or not, give each child 200 seconds a day, too. Refrain from paying the bills or swapping office stories on the phone with Bill when your kid hands you the highlight of his life, his flying cockroach. Family events are perfect occasions for giving your kids the legacy of the wellthy investments you want them to inherit, a legacy far more useful than your money.

Reserve Club 200 seconds for your lover, too; and think diversity. Invent pet names for each other, but try again if moose and snoopy come to mind. Jump in the shower with aerosol cans of whipped cream or smear each other with honey to lick off. Send the kids and the babysitter to a double feature with ice cream cone money to keep them out of the house a bit longer. After you lock the doors and close the blinds, make love in the hall closet or any place you never do it. You'll have no regrets until your mom uses her key to open the front door, ready to take you Venus fly trapping.

Men, remember the dates of your anniversary and her birthday and bring her one rose every day for a week to celebrate each of them. Women, write "I love you" in lipstick on the bottom of the toilet seat he always leaves up. Tell why you find each other sexy and what you liked about the other when you first met. Trade hugs, kisses, and compliments any time of day. "The meat loaf was particularly tasty" or "I admire the way you took charge at the parent meeting tonight" are chicken steps that can be taken daily, as opposed to once-a-year flowers. However, you might want to consider "I adore you, Mabel" flashing in purple neon on a theater marquis. We are particularly partial to the latter. A less expensive way to be romantic is to spend your Club 200 seconds chatting, especially when you echo his/her feelings instead of rehearsing your next sentence. Never forget these chicken steps. These steps work especially well in refining our rediscovered intimacy with our life partners.

Learn that "selfish" is not a dirty word. Many of us give all our time away to our children, our spouses, and our work. They don't appreciate it and you won't have the Club 200 time you need to invest in "self" and in your spouse that is so necessary to keep a wellthy balance.

Sad Sally was distraught. She had been married 28 years. Her life was perfect: perfect husband, perfect children, perfect home in a perfect community. They did almost everything together. Everything was devoted to family: taking Jimmy here, Fran there, little Sally elsewhere. Ball games, soccer, recitals, birthday parties, school plays, music, it was perfect. Sad Sally can't stop crying. Her perfect husband left her today, said he didn't know her. The kids had grown up and moved away. Their heavy investment in the kids had left their marriage account bankrupt. They no longer knew each other. Invest carefully in all of your funds!

Draw out your bubbles (roles) using the example below. Make the size of the bubble represent its importance to you. The overlap should represent how much time you spend with that part of your life. Now, color them to represent how they make you feel. How well invested are you? Where do you need to spend more time and effort? Which bubbles represent positive investments and which are draining? Sometimes, this exercise is too difficult to do on your own.

Sad Sally found her bubbles were impossible to draw. Sally turned to a psychologist for help. A psychologist often is invaluable in helping to restore balance to a wellthy account gone bad. We wholeheartedly recommend assessing each segment of your wellthy account on a regular basis and reviewing your assessments with your physician, counselor, clergy, and others qualified consultants to maximize your wellth.

While books and websites can help you get along with other people, most overlook one of the most gratifying aspects of peopl-ease. It is sharing part of your self when you aren't required to do so, otherwise known as the "Giving Fund." Successful and wellthy retirees said that one of the 3 things they would do differently if they could repeat their lives would be to spend more time in activities that made a difference. Next to sex and cotton candy, what is more wondrous than the smile on a hospitalized child's face when you dance around in a clown suit? Or the way an elderly person's face brightens as she strokes the kitten you put in her lap? In many areas, volunteer bureaus maintain a broad menu of organizations eager to receive your time and efforts. It's best to sign up for activities compatible with your talents, be they delivering books to the homebound, raising funds for a shelter, or collecting native plant seeds to beautify your community. If you enjoy writing, compose news releases or manage a home page for your cause. Like kids? Be a homework tutor, big brother, or foster grandma. Want something more active? Get in shape for a charity run, lead a booster club, play Saturday softball with the kids. A simple way to share your bubble is to be kind to your garbage dump. Show everyone who will stand still how you use plastic bags at least twice, recycle everything that doesn't holler, and take an extra minute to compost left-over veggies. Conserving your environment is the ultimate charity because it benefits everyone both today and tomorrow. Adopt a local roadway with neighbors and get the bonus of strengthening friendships and getting more fit. Look for birds in a park, plant trees on parkways, hoe a community garden, or work your own backyard. Use flushable kitty litter and earth-friendly detergent. Check with your children for umpteen more ways to improve the wellth of your surroundings. Practice pleasing the people who mean the most to you. Doing so will help you with the tricky business of balancing your many roles, not to mention your life.

CHAPTER 12. BALANCING YOUR INVESTMENTS

Financease, foodease, fitease, and self/peoplease form a pyramid in which each part is perfectly balanced by the other three. If any one component weakens, the pyramid begins to crumble. The cornerstone of the pyramid is physical health, since it's difficult to lead a balanced life when we are weak, obese, or sick; and lugging an oxygen tank spoils the view. Yet, most of us spend most of our time making the most money possible, while our bodies get the leftovers a gerbil would sneer at. It seems that maintaining our health is like a paper cut on our thumb: we pay no attention to our thumb until it hurts. Certainly, financease to provide adequate nutrition, medical care, and safety is essential, as is feeling good about ourselves and getting along with most other people. We strive constantly to balance the components of our wellth, in part because they fluctuate from day to day and decade to decade, sometimes wildly, all our lives. The best way to balance our wellth budget is called income averaging in the financial world, defined as making small, repetitive deposits in investment funds, deposits that, over time, soften extreme swings in the market. Using this system, an investor with $600.00 to stash, deposits $50.00 in his account each month for a year rather than in one lump sum. When we make small, daily contributions to each component of our wellth, we gain the wellth we need to sustain us through hard times. The wellth of each account expands and shrinks with age and life events, such as marriage, divorce, job changes, and the arrival or departure of children. We would dance on tabletops if we could be forever healthy, wealthy, and wise, as well as gorgeous, smart, and supremely happy. We can waltz just as gracefully and successfully when we march in chicken steps toward our mini goals in each area of wellth.

For example, we enrich our personal lives and polish our people skills when we make little contributions to our accounts the same way we earned nutrition and fitness body bucks. Even a wisp of time pays off. You might learn 5 new words, compose a serenade, or sing it to a special person within your 200 seconds a day of both selfease and peoplease time. Or you could exercise your brain by memorizing a new haiku every day, while you strengthen your psyche by meditating with them. You would learn a new language 200 seconds at a time if you kept at it for 5 years. Staying fit, eating nutritious meals, stashing money, and reserving time for yourself and the people important to you spells balance. When a serious illness, death, or divorce occurs, most of us do what we must without worrying about our Club 200. If you have made wise investments in your wellthy account, you will weather the storm better. If you respond appropriately, you will maintain balance. It's healthy to grieve about terrible events, including the death of your dog. Your sadness may even bolster your selfease by demonstrating that you can cope with loss, so that the next setback won't loom quite as large. You may find that exercise helps relieve the stress associated with your loss, further strengthening your fitease assets. Unfortunately, during times of sadness and loss, many individuals' foodease accounts diminish rapidly and, following our model, cause damage to their selfease. We strongly recommend that you allow yourself the time to heal, then slowly step back to wellth.

Everyone loves Laughing Lana. She's the life of the party who breaks up her friends with her crazy jokes, especially the cracks about her girth. Lana is too busy nurturing her family and friends to save any money. Her motto is "Eat, drink, and be merry; for tomorrow, we diet." By never exercising beyond walking to the fridge, Lana weighs 280 pounds and suffers from hypertension, diabetes, and leg ulcers. She didn't laugh when warned that she faced a premature death unless she began to balance her nutrition and fitness accounts with her people-pleasing skills. Despite her health problems, she had what Big Bucks Bob can only long for, a selfease that Native American Inuits call "nuannaapog", which means taking extravagant pleasure in being alive. Bob is 62 and lives on $150,000 a year in dividends from his investments. He is proud that his children will inherit a generous legacy. Meanwhile, he lugs his medical charts between his homes in Arizona and Florida where he spends $500.00 a month for medications, apart from the bills for his surgeries and convalescences. He loves his ice cream, chocolate anything, and says it won't help his health to quit smoking at his age. Because he insists on existing with emphysema, diabetes, and hardening of the arteries,

Bob finds very little joy in being alive. His foodease component is shaking his pyramid to pieces with earthquake force.

Lana and Bob may not be able to overcome all the damage they've done to their health, but they can improve the quality of their lives by refining, in small steps, their eating and exercise habits. They can also leave their children the gift of good health practices, an inheritance far more valuable than witty jokes and vacation homes. You may be asking, "I want to protect my health, but how can chicken stepping be any fun? I like to enjoy myself in my free time. And I don't want to give up everything I love to improve my body." The best answer we know is that financial investing may require giving up $10.00 a day for a future million dollars. Is it reasonable to give up a burrito at lunch today for a winter retreat in the Tropics a few years down the road? Your answer is probably yes; the burrito for the winter retreat trade is definitely worth it. Investing in your body requires sacrifices of time, but you reap the reward and pleasure of playing volleyball or working in the garden. It requires giving up a second helping of deep-dish pizza or that after-dinner cigarette; but, in return, you can fit into that slinky outfit only your daughter used to be able to wear and you have the breath to dance all night. Are these sacrifices significant when they make the difference between occupying a healthy body and a gravesite?

"But," you may counter, "how does the average mortal like me find the time to invest money prudently, eat judiciously, exercise productively, spend private time, family time, and lover time every day, and still volunteer on my day off?" It's not as impossible as it seems when you make each activity serve double or triple duty. A clever timewrap is to get paid for doing something you are so passionate about that you would do it for nothing if you won the lottery. A chef, social worker, teacher, or astronomer whose enthusiasm inspires colleagues and students to do their best is most likely well-vested in selfease and peoplease. A dedicated painter, geneticist, homemaker, or computer whiz who also trains for marathons is so wellthy he/she doesn't need this book. In your work life, don't expect to feel inspired every hour of every day; but, if you're a nervous wreck or an angry troll at the end of most workdays, stop tearing down your pyramid and find another job. Killing yourself for money is too absurd to consider, no matter how many of us persist in doing it.

How much time are we talking about anyway? You might minimize the time you spend on your finances by arranging for automatic payroll or checking account contributions to your funds. To streamline grocery store time and temptation, plan nutritious menus and shop once a week when you aren't starving. Your daily fitease time is too important to skip, considering it's a trivial 5 % of the 10-hour day most of us spend working and commuting. To make it a habit, insist on doing a little each day even if it's less than ½ hour. Cross your heart and hope to die, or timewrap it with your private or family time. Devoting 3 1/3 minutes a day to our partner or kids may seem ludicrously brief; but it isn't, given that the average couple converses only ½ hour a week. Mostly, they chat about intimate topics, such as "Did you pick up the dog's suit from the cleaners or give the hamster a bath?" Likewise, we may take more time brushing our teeth than communicating with our children. Spending 200 seconds per child, times an average of 2 per household, plus 200 seconds more with your partner, adds up to the astronomical total of 10 minutes a day devoted to the people we purport to value the most. We should be compulsive about it, despite the sink full of dirty dishes or dust bunnies under the bed.

We've mentioned ways to wrap foodease and fitease activities around self- and peoplease, as in family hikes at the zoo, picnic lunch included. Hiring your teenagers and all their friends helps get the job done when you stuff them with endless pizza and blast them with rock music. You might haul the gang to the mall and turn your teens loose among the video games while you and your partner walk, talk, and slurp up a raspberry smoothie with 2 straws. Garnish your family outings with a couple of hours per month teaching handicapped children to bat a softball or tutoring kids in English, and you've mixed a wonderfully balanced investment cocktail. What a bargain it is, yielding 200 more bucks a day of ease for an hour of your time, as follows:

1. 30 minutes fitease/selfease/family time
2. 10 minutes family time
3. 5 minutes community service time per day for 2 hours a month
4. 15 minutes family/foodease = ONE little hour, total

Timewraps are great diversifiers, too. For example, devoting all your free time to your golf score or the football game contributes neither balance nor variety to your life. The same is true of clinging like a moth to your home computer or camping in the SUV so that you can chauffeur the kids to endless soccer games and band practice. Children need private time the same as you do; they can misplace their selfness when every minute of their day is programmed, the same as you. Intersperse virtual reality friends with companions that breathe and sneeze after you close the websites and browse a real flea market. Shock everyone by leaving the house to shoot baskets or check out a library book instead of clicking your mouse. You'll be refreshed by the novelty of playing a difficult chess match or hiking up a 5 degree grade. We'll forgive you if you email us once in a while with Timewraps that work for you and check the Wellthy site for more ideas from other readers.

Balance is relative. When you feel good physically and emotionally and like most of your "self" most of the time, your accounts are probably well balanced. You have wellth when you are physically and mentally active, believe you have the best job for you, and the people you love aren't trying to beam you out of the galaxy. Life is a voyage we take just once. The wellthy life is hoisting the anchor high over the deck and sailing around the world for the sheer adventure of the trip, raging storms, becalmed seas, and all. May your voyage be filled with **life, joy, and happiness**.

There is, of course, one final account that you must pay attention to during your voyage to "Wellth." Your "Spiritual Account" is the glue that holds everything together. Invest heavily and often! Because of the intensely personal nature of our spiritual selves, this arena is best examined within your own religious and/or spiritual community and is beyond the scope of this book. However, this journey can follow our chicken step approach by investing often and in small steps always seeking enlightenment.

30 MORE WAYS TO EASE INTO EATING

1. When you eat less, you'll lose weight. When you eat better, you'll lose weight.
2. Imagine that you are thin. What are you doing instead of eating?
3. Pay the kids a dime every time they catch you standing up and eating.
4. Ask yourself, "Do I really need to eat this or can I wait for something I do want?"
5. Eat dinner naked in front of a full-length mirror.
6. Prepare a meal featuring the kids' school colors.
7. Toast cumin seeds in a frying pan and inhale the aroma.
8. Picnic in each of the kids' bedrooms; yours, too, if you are brave.
9. Anything deep-fried can be oven baked, even fried chicken.
10. Prepare mashed potatoes with broth, not butter.
11. Simmer sliced onions in balsamic vinegar with a bit of sugar.

12. Make fruit butters with fresh fruit pulp and a little sugar.
13. Grocery shop after you have eaten.
14. Prepare canapés from around the world and invent new ones.
15. Stuff kale leaves with kasha and raisins; poach in tomato juice.
16. Fill cabbage leaves with tuna; simmer in chicken stock.
17. Stuff grape leaves with rice and toasted pine nuts.
18. Pack red peppers with corn or other vegetables.
19. Wrap lettuce leaves around low-fat cream cheese and veggies.
20. Make crudities with pre-cut veggies and low-cal sauce for dipping.
21. Present Greek antipasto with olives, feta cheese, and roasted peppers.
22. Wrap thinly sliced proscuitto around melon balls.
23. Grill low fat hot dogs chunks on skewers with veggies or marshmallows.
24. Whip up a fluffy omelet with 6 whites, 3 yolks, and 1 tsp baking powder.
25. Serve a cold gazpacho or hot egg-drop soup.
26. Poach fake eggs in tomato cups.
27. Have a holiday and disaster plan.
28. Whittle away at the bad stuff, one ¼ serving at a time.
29. In a restaurant, fill the doggie bag before you eat.
30. Learn to love something else.

Always remember, don't deny yourself anything, but eat it sparingly.

25 MORE WAYS TO GET FIT

1. When you're stuck in traffic, suck in your gut and hold for a three count, relax, repeat.
2. Tighten your abs 10 times when you're watching the tube.
3. Stretch up to the sky on tiptoes, as far as you can reach.
4. Plan how to look irresistibly sexy at your next tryst with your partner.
5. Imagine you are very fit. What do you look like?
6. Lift your knees and rotate your ankles seated at your desk.
7. Press your palms, arms, and elbows together waiting in the car.
8. Do 10 slow half squats at home when you're put on hold.
9. Squeeze your glutei while waiting for anything.
10. Go to the store and try on swimsuits. Do you like what you see?
11. Walk a big dog.
12. Take the stairs double time.
13. Unhunch and lean backwards at your desk.
14. Swing and teeter totter with or without the kids.

15. Practice a new dance step.
16. Toss a Frisbee for the dog or cockatoo to catch.
17. Extend your arms backwards with bent elbows.
18. Stretch your neck, rotating your head from side to side.
19. Go fly a kite.
20. Breathe deeply twice and hold a short time. Repeat.
21. Take a walk with your partner.
22. Fidget a lot (the British call it otching); some people use worry beads.
23. With arms at your sides and thumbs pointed backwards, suck in your belly button.
24. Plan a new outfit for the fit you.
25. Buy a well-made pair of athletic shoes that fit you.

Remember, a bad investment is costly. Chickenstepping to fitease helps prevent injury! The rules have changed: "Pain, No Gain."

25 MORE WAYS TO SELFEASE

1. Pet a friendly animal.
2. Teach a kid to fly a kite.
3. Buy yourself a rose.
4. Scream and holler at a ball game.
5. Cuddle a baby.
6. Look up at the clouds or the stars for 5 minutes.
7. Throw a paper airplane.
8. Feed the birds and squirrels.
9. Compliment someone.
10. Play Pat-a-Cake with a toddler.
11. Sing a silly song.
12. Recite a limerick.
13. Visit the zoo.
14. Read a poem.
15. Plant a tree.
16. Learn a new joke.
17. Eat popcorn at a movie matinee (skip the butter).
18. Email or write a faraway friend.

19. Wear a happy face in the supermarket.
20. Look at a work of art for 5 minutes.
21. Listen to a melodic piece of classical music.
22. Phone home.
23. Sample different colognes at the drug store.
24. Visit a new site on the Internet.
25. Play with a child.

We invite you to tell us how you maintain your ease and we'll plan to publish the appropriate ones.

APPENDIX A

Timewrap

You've heard of time-warps (doing two things at once) and may be convinced you occupy one because you can't borrow a minute, much less half an hour, for yourself. Think of time-wraps to overcome the warps and hunt for ways to make your time do double duty.

1. At doctors' offices, including the family doc, orthodontist, and optometrist's office, walk out when your child disappears into a back cubicle and walk a flight or 2 of stairs. If there aren't any stairs, patter down the sidewalk outside.
2. Get out of your minivan while waiting for the kids to win their games and dash up and down the sidelines, cheering for your team.
3. Ditto for car camping while they finish choir practice, piano lessons, ballet class, and school play rehearsal . . .
4. While you're on the cell phone listening to your long-winded aunt Mabel, make a list of things to do tomorrow. It avoids going shopping and forgetting the item you went for. Sometimes.
5. Activate your crock-pot and have your dinner ready when you get home from work.

6. Use your microwave oven for more than defrosting. It's easy to prepare entire meals in half an hour while you feed the dog.
7. Ask the children to feed the dog. Children helping out at home is a fine idea despite the battles.
8. When you cook, make enough for 2 evenings and keep trying for 4. Labeling and dating the contents avoids a freezer full of mystery meat and freezer burn.
9. Dr. P's grandfather posted a list of Greek or Latin words on the toilet paper every day and insisted we kids learn them.
10. We also had to recite Frost's poetry when we drove in New England and repeat the Latin names of plants and trees we saw.

ACKNOWLEDGEMENTS

This project has been a work-in-progress for more years than I want to count. I started developing the concept of "Wellthy" as I saw what happened to so many of my patients as they lost their health but were such astute businessmen and women. I thank them for their stories. I thank them for teaching me what I needed to teach them. I thank the staff at Lake Zurich Family Treatment Center, past and present, for all of their hard work, for everything they do to make my life easier so I can be in the room treating patients and for everything they do for each and every patient who comes into our office.

There are some people in my life who make me truly "Wellthy." The ones who always remind me that I'm not perfect are my children. I am blessed to have five children; but I was lucky only to have to put three of them through college. Two came through marriage after college. Erin, Jeremy, Lisa, Tim, and Allyson are my major "Wellthy" accounts. One of the dividends of married children is grandchildren, and Jackson and Hannah are the gifts that keep giving. My mother,

Bette Segal, and my father-in-law, Bernard Rafal, have always been there for me, no matter what. It's always nice to know who's in your corner. To my brothers and sisters, Alan, Abe, Robert, Brian, Bernie, Annabelle, Linda, Susan, Dale, Martha, Chris, and Nancy, I thank them for being such a wonderful part of my life. They comprise another "Wellthy" account that is well-funded and I know this account will continue to grow and support me forever.

To Barbara Phillips, Ph.D., my co-author, many thanks for the many years she has put into this project along with me. Her humor and vast knowledge of the world and writing helped translate my concept from thought to print.

Lastly, I'd like to thank my wife, Renee, for sharing her life with me. She wears many hats, including lover, partner, best friend, confidant, mother, bubbe, Practice Administrator, editor; and she always has "my back." I thank her for each hat she wears. She makes me truly "Wellthy!"

Thank you all for adding so much to my life!
Stewart Segal, MD

www.ingramcontent.com/pod-product-compliance
Lightning Source LLC
Chambersburg PA
CBHW050131280326
41933CB00010B/1335

* 9 7 8 0 6 1 5 5 3 8 0 7 5 *